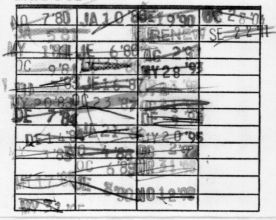

The Female Fix

The Female Fix

tình trạng, trắc trở, khó khăn

Muriel Nellis

Houghton Mifflin Company Boston 1980

Library of Congress Cataloging in Publication Data
Nellis, Muriel.
    The female fix.

    1. Drugs and women — United States. 2. Alcohol and women — United States. I. Title.
HV5824.W6N44   362.2'93   79-23971
ISBN 0-395-27786-8

Printed in the United States of America

S 10 9 8 7 6 5 4 3 2 1

The author is grateful for permission to quote from FROM HERE TO ETERNITY, by James Jones. Reprinted by permission of Charles Scribner's Sons and Collins Publishers. Copyright 1951 James Jones.

TO JOE,
my devoted best friend, my most important
personal choice, my colleague, my husband.

Acknowledgments

A book, like a painting, is the visible result of impressions earlier absorbed. This expression of many prisms of light and color was shared with me by hundreds of women who serve others, some by their work, others by will. They cannot be named — some because they abide by a group decision of anonymity, others because they fear punishing consequences for past mistakes. I trust that I have served their friendship well.

Alberta Henderson labored in arid bureaucratic soil and planted the only sturdy seed of professional commitment for drug-dependent women. Her unique perseverance was vital to my work in this field.

The concern and energy of the participants at the first National Forum on Drugs, Alcohol, and Women, in 1975, evidenced the public, private, and professional desire to confront the problems addressed by the conference. The immediate and continuing attention to the plight of addicted women by then First Lady Betty Ford, by House Judiciary Committee chairman Peter W. Rodino (D–N.J.), and by Paul Rogers (D–Fla.) raised this unrecognized need to national prominence and lent it the weight of law.

For Forum support and extended assistance beyond 1975, thanks to Leslie Maddox, Betti Pate, Virginia Essex, Lauren Sullivan, and a stalwart team associated with Miami-Dade Rehabilitative Services. Continuity of friendship and mutual purpose has enriched my palette.

I am grateful for special fidelity and direction from many state and regional members of the dynamic Alliance on Drugs, Alcohol, and Women's Health, whose efforts were publicly heralded by Congresswoman Corinne (Lindy) Boggs (D–La.), a gracious ally.

For long-valued counsel and criticism, my gratitude to Mary Hager. Frank J. Vocci (FDA–Bureau of Drugs) generously provided scientific insight and interpretation. Ann Buchwald's faith and wisdom were moving forces in getting this novice to confront the empty paper. Austin Olney made me a believer in serendipity, while Helena Bentz kept me faithful to precision. For shape and texture, the skills of my editor, Frances Tenenbaum, were mighty tools.

Finally, to all the people I call family, I am thankful for that most personal element of experience called feelings, which lend the tone to every endeavor.

Contents

The Female Fix

Long before this book was written it was lived—
by many women—who are any one of us.

1

The Unadmitted Problem

FOR TOO LONG, the lonely anguish of women's drug and alcohol habits has been the subject of whispered confidences, gossip-column innuendoes, and hushed family embarrassment. For too long, this anguish has been viewed as an individual fall from grace. Admittedly, every situation is distinguished, in some way, from any other. These differences confirm the uniqueness of human experience, but they do not change a universal fact: an insidious epidemic has been raging among the women of this nation — addiction to drugs. All kinds of drugs, in tablets, capsules, and liquids — tranquilizers, sleeping pills, diet pills, pain killers, alcohol — over-the-counter and prescribed. And all of them legal. The combinations are literally mind boggling.

In 1978, the acting director of the National Institute on Drug Abuse told the House Select Committee on Narcotics Abuse and Control that, in the past year, 36 million women had used tranquilizers; 16 million used sedatives (sleeping pills); 12 million used stimulants primarily in the form of diet pills; and almost 12 million women received prescriptions for these drugs from doctors for the first time. Those numbers do not include whole classes of prescribed pain killers, all of which are mood altering and addictive. Nor do they include the billions of doses dispensed to patients directly, without a prescription, in doctors' offices, in military, public, or private hospitals, and in clinics or nursing homes. Nor do these statistics tell us how many of these women used combinations of prescription drugs or combined them with the most widely used depressant, alcohol. According to recent figures, at least half of the probably 10 million alcoholics in the country are women.

Social Stigma

For women, legal drug and alcohol abuse has become a common hazard that threatens one out of every four of us. The least suspecting among us is the most vulnerable. Elaine, like many other women, spent years trying to deny that she was dependent on drugs. She explained:

> It's hell for a woman to admit a drug habit. It's frightening too. I think most women on drugs or alcohol bear a heavier load of guilt and anger than men. A man on drugs may not get respect, but he can usually find some lady to care for him. We don't even have that to count on. A woman with a drug need is the lowest; she has not one single attribute that society values. And we feel so personally guilty. We blame ourselves; our men also blame us. And when we look outside for help, most professionals blame us too.

Since the social stigma associated with alcohol or drug use is particularly severe for women, it is all the more difficult for millions of women to confront this agonizing fact of life, even though it is a poorly kept secret. Writing about women and alcoholism, Joseph Hirsh offered the following insight on the cultural underpinnings of the existing social stigma:

> Women represent important social and moral symbols that are the bedrock of society. And when angels fall, they fall disturbingly far. We would rather have them in their place; which is another way of saying that they define and make our own place possible and even more comfortable.

We learn and are reminded that, as females, our actions affect the social, moral, and inspirational symbols of civilized behavior. We are our great-grandmothers' posterity. The responsibilities of tradition either invade or enrich our inner and outer lives, depending on whether or not meeting those expectations is perceived as oppressive or fulfilling.

It would follow that an imperfect cornerstone in the structure of our society is uncomfortable, even threatening. Generally, and individually, there has been a disinclination to consider, let alone accept, the existence of women addicts. Even now, that turn-away mentality persists.

A few days after Betty Ford, with her customary candor, admitted her addiction to alcohol and drugs, I was invited to lunch at a suburban country club. Everyone touched by the news media was now aware of Mrs. Ford's previously well-guarded agony. Would her forthright courage be the master key, I wondered, that would finally unlock the door of secrecy, open a public dialogue, and clear the way for other women in quietly desperate trouble to seek help? In celebration of the possible new dawn of women's health, I accepted the luncheon invitation. In tune with the season, I was bursting with anticipation. On this traditionally "distaff" day at the clubhouse, the scent of freshly groomed new grass was laced with Norell, Chanel, Arpège, and salon hair-spray mists, heightening my image of healthy people enjoying good care. But my sense of well-being was sharply altered when I heard:

"I don't think Mrs. Ford had any right to embarrass her family."

"Right. If she had a problem, she should have kept it to herself."

"Irresponsible! Some things are no one else's business. She ought to know that better than others. What kind of example is she?"

"It's so selfish — and damned confusing."

Hardly pausing to greet my lunch mates, I quickly proposed that Mrs. Ford's public admission might be of critical comfort to other similarly wounded women; that they might feel less isolation and self-loathing and might even consider admitting the need for help. There was loud, instant disagreement from everyone.

I listened with dismay as these articulate women carefully put a safe distance between themselves and both the bad news and Mrs. Ford, the messenger who carried it. Neither was welcome.

But, welcome or not, Betty Ford *is* critical to this issue. Because of her special status in the life of this country, her extraordinary admission compels an open examination of all the dimensions of this commonplace problem, including the old labels and myths. It must now be made clear: Women who get "hooked" on drugs are not necessarily poor creatures who live on the fringe, outside the mainstream of American life. If a former First Lady, proper congressional wife, and devoted mother could entrust herself to treatment for addiction, then that affliction can no longer be viewed as just the disease of disreputable women. Nice ladies get messed up too.

Moreover, the very nature of Betty Ford's life experience exemplifies the stressful demands made on the lives of many millions of other nurturing, hard-working women. The arena of visibility is only different in degree. Even the wife who enjoys sharing the challenge of her husband's ambitious pursuits is required to make constant, personal sacrifices on the altar of his career, be it political, military, corporate, or academic. Whatever the milieu, personal and family needs must be secondary, must adapt. Lifestyles, friends, and activities are often determined more by his colleague's expectations than by her choice. On the job, male attitudes still define the relationships between men and women, and male criteria circumscribe the success of women — married or single. The appearance of proper behavior is necessary, whether or not it produces frustration, anxiety, or loneliness. The rules of the road exact a heavy toll.

Who can blame my luncheon friends, or yours, for instinctively trying to dissociate themselves from unsettling realities? There is an inherent desire to affirm traditions. The greater the chance of identification with characteristics considered negative by society, the faster the need to repulse the thought. Betty Ford defied the predictability of the social order by humanizing it. Inevitably, that means recognizing frailties as well as potential strengths.

Her statement raises other questions. Ostensibly Mrs. Ford had the best medical care this country could provide. If she could become accidentally addicted, are any of the rest of us safe from possible damage from "safe and efficacious" drugs? In fact, how many of us are already chemical cripples? Would we or anyone else know? What is "over medication"? Why is it insidious and dangerous? Are women more vulnerable? Why? When? And what is being done about any of it?

The Pattern of Prescription-Drug Use

While it is now clear that women as well as men are pursuing dangerous drug-using paths, health specialists and official regulators continue to focus on a male drug culture. This presumably benign oversight has permitted a malignant growth to go unchecked. But neither ignorance nor denial will alter the facts.

Statistics attesting to the enormity of the patterns of prescription-drug use by women are shocking. Of the 160 million prescriptions written last year for tranquilizers, sedatives, and stimulants, only about 10 percent were authorized by psychiatrists, the one group of doctors whose training emphasizes the effects of psychoactive therapeutics. The largest percentage of these prescriptions was written by general practitioners, internists, and obstetricians-gynecologists. Depending on the drug classification — tranquilizer, sedative, or stimulant — 60 to 80 percent of all the drugs prescribed were for female patients.

During each of the past several years, 90 percent of the women seen in hospitals for drug-related emergencies used legal, prescribed drugs; and the greatest number of drug-related deaths were the result of a combination of drugs plus alcohol.

Mental health experts estimate that about 10 percent of our population suffers from some serious mental disease, but that almost three-quarters of the nation is affected by disabling anxiety, insecurity, tension — the totality of the pressures of living. They further speculate that 70 to 80 percent of the symptoms of illness told to physicians, from sleeplessness to stomach aches, are but the open wounds of hidden life strains — an acceptable way to present pleas for relief.

This national malaise has particular significance for women, as the following facts indicate:

• At every age over 15, more women than men receive treatment for mental health problems. Except in the 25 to 34-year range, the institutional diagnosis of "depression" is far greater for women than men. (This greater female proportion, seen at hospitals and clinics, does not include those who are similarly treated by general practitioners, private mental-health therapists, religious counselors, self-help groups, or those troubled but untreated.)

• Women make the majority of visits to doctors. They have higher rates of admission to general hospitals and report more physical ailments.

• In addition, women enter and return to private psychiatric therapy in and outside of hospitals more often than men.

• Minimally, women are prescribed *more than twice* the amount of drugs than are men, *for the same psychological symptoms.*

• Although women of almost every description are represented in this emotionally distressed group, single women present the fewest symptoms of mental disorder; married women with families, the greatest number.

• A sizable percentage of women who finally seek help for emotional problems have already turned to alcohol or mood-affecting drugs for stress therapy.

• In the past ten years, the number of women who voluntarily sought help for alcoholism has doubled, though still not approaching the 5 million females presumed to be alcoholic. The number of deaths from cirrhosis of the liver is rapidly increasing among women.

Although there is a tendency within the health bureaucracy — and therefore the literature — to define dependence on mood-altering drugs separately from dependence on drugs prescribed for a specific physical symptom, questions are being raised increasingly about the validity of this distinction. What may begin as a purely medical therapy too often becomes an addictive problem.

Another traditional distinction without a difference between drugs and medications bears some comment. To differentiate between the so-called hard and soft drugs, implying degrees of damage, it has become professionally fashionable to refer to physical and psychological addictions as dissimilar. Those women who have suffered stomach cramps, nervous perspiration, or irritability at either the thought, or the absence, of their customary drink or dose, strongly disagree with these arbitrary variations. A more realistic definition of addiction presumes that all function is intertwined.

Even to distinguish between addictive drugs by using the words *hard* and *soft* — like *major* and *minor* — promote the drawing of improper inferences regarding their destructive potential. Children born to mothers addicted to opiates frequently suffer immediate trauma that may cause long-term consequences. Likewise, the growing population of limbless, brain-damaged, facially disfigured, or motor-impaired children is evidence of the inherent dangers associated with maternal use of tranquilizers, sedatives, and alcohol.

At the Conference of Pain, Discomfort, and Humanitarian Care, recently held at the National Institutes of Health, many speakers concluded that the management of chronic pain has become a major problem, affecting as much as 40 percent of all Americans. Such common diseases as arthritis, gout, back pains, headaches, and rheumatism are costing sufferers not only pain, but billions of dollars each year, largely for ineffective treatment, much of it in the form of addictive drugs.

It appears that too many doctors are responding to, "It doesn't matter what's causing it, just help." They are helping by prescribing more drugs and, in some cases, causing new problems. Specialists in pain clinics are openly concerned by the apparent absence of understanding among general practitioners of the peculiar and unpleasant interactions between different pain relievers. Similarly, among behavioral specialists there is great consternation over the simultaneous prescription of sedatives with pain drugs, which often promote serious physical and emotional depression.

Sadly, the history of progress in drug development is spotty and repetitious. Too often a new discovery is no more than a variation on an older, troublesome theme. Just as heroin was perceived as an alternative treatment for morphine addiction, now methadone is the (addictive) substitute for heroin. The "major" tranquilizers, correctly hailed as reducing the use of electroconvulsive shock treatments or brain surgery in severe psychotic disturbance, are now overprescribed for traumas and neurotic conditions that would never have required or been treated by the earlier, dramatic procedures. In the same continuum of reduced risk, barbiturates and other heavy sedatives were replaced by the so-called minor tranquilizers. But this breakthrough foisted more of these drugs on larger populations — for a wider variety of milder nondisease conditions.

Once again, new research, new remedies. New choices, new consequences. Increasing combinations are increasingly harmful. Some are lethal. The most serious problem we confront is not so much with any one drug, which, when taken wisely and prescribed carefully, may be very helpful, but rather with the growing numbers of compounds and variations of the same chemical classes, and the range of professionals empowered to dispense them.

"Minor" Tranquilizers—Major Hazard

To many physicians and patients, with little or no understanding of severe brain or mental disorders, "minor" tranquilizers are equated with mild ones, and *mild* sounds safe. Safe tranquilizers? Not on your life. True, there is virtually no drug that is completely safe, and certainly not for everyone. But this class of drugs, which comes in so many colors, bearing so many names, so freely prescribed for so many types and degrees of misery, is full of guile and without innocence.

Recently, Dr. David Smith, Director of the Haight-Ashbury Clinic in San Francisco, noted that withdrawal symptoms occurred in people who had taken only low, therapeutic doses of Valium for more than a year. (Valium is the single most prescribed drug in the United States.) Although former alcoholics seemed especially predisposed to this withdrawal reaction, persons without a history of alcoholism were also affected. Doris had such an experience.

> For five years after my first introduction to tranquilizers I used them daily. Not in large amounts, but regularly. First I took one for a way to sleep — when my head was so full of problems, and the noise of thinking kept me awake. After that, I just took them to prevent anything from "getting to me." When my fourteen-year-old daughter asked me for one before a big test, I decided to get rid of the pills. I was miserable, my nerves were shot, and I felt like I had a virus — exhausted, then aching and tense. It took between two and three months before I felt normal.

As drugs proliferate and medical care becomes increasingly fragmented, overprescription becomes commonplace — and too easy to blame on the other guy. In surveys taken among doctors about overprescribing patterns, the respondents overwhelmingly indicate concern about "other doctors" who engage in the practice, but deny subscribing to that behavior themselves. As one doctor told me, "There are bad apples in any profession. The rest of us aren't responsible for them. That's a job for the authorities; it has nothing to do with me. I seldom use more than a couple dozen medications in my practice. I'm a specialist, and the hundreds of other compounds don't mean much to me."

Alas, they often mean *too* much to the patient who consults more than one specialist, including my good friend Kathy.

Just prior to starting a new job, Kathy went to her internist for a routine physical. She mentioned that she had heard that her new boss had a reputation as a perfectionist, and she admitted feeling some anxiety about it. Her doctor prescribed a mild, low-dose tranquilizer, just to get her "over the hump."

During her first week at work, Kathy strained a muscle

in her neck. Since it was quite painful, an office mate sent Kathy to her own neurologist, who prescribed a "muscle relaxant." A week or so later, a totally unrelated condition, some ovary spasms, led Kathy to her gynecologist, who prescribed a third medication.

What Kathy didn't know until the reaction set in was that all three prescriptions contained different amounts of the same kind of tranquilizer.

> They all looked different. They each had separate instructions. Each doctor was satisfied that I was healthy, except for some minor discomfort. Aside from asking about any allergies or family history of major diseases, they never questioned me about drugs.

Fortunately, Kathy's reaction to these drugs was paradoxical. Instead of becoming overly tranquilized, her behavior reversed, and her otherwise pleasant and friendly disposition turned curt and short-tempered. Out of common concern over this disquieting, uncharacteristic behavior, a group of long-time friends gathered to find out what was troubling her and to offer their help. She was astonished. She had no idea that her personality had been so affected. Together, Kathy and her friends traced the events that seemed to coincide with her erratic moods, and only then did the pattern of drug use emerge. It soon became clear that there was a relationship between her behavior and her visits to doctors, each followed by a new prescription.

Kathy did not know the active ingredients of the drugs prescribed, so she and a friend drove to the pharmacy that had sold her all three. They requested copies of the manufacturers' description circulars that accompany the drugs supplied to pharmacists. Since there were no instructions from the doctors to withhold such information, surrendering the inserts was only a minor inconvenience to the druggist. Although the language of the pamphlets seemed undecipherable at first, it soon made her puzzling behavior clear. Somewhere in the small print Kathy found her own symptoms.

The circulars warned that "careful consideration should be given to the pharmacology of other psychotropics employed, which may potentiate the action of Valium." There might be "adverse reactions": "headaches," "constipation," "tremors." She had experienced them all. The pamphlets had a name for other behaviors she had shown: "paradoxical reactions." Examples of these included "acute hyperexcited states," "anxiety," "insomnia," and "rage." Kathy had mistakenly attributed her symptoms to her job and some physical demons.

Even if many physicians sincerely believe that the drugs they prescribe are not toxic, one cannot attribute similar naiveté to the industry that produces them and markets them, through the doctor, to the patient-consumer. I actually heard the head of a major medical advertising company describe how his company, through artful language and marketing campaigns, has helped "enlarge the whole concept of illness" in order to accommodate the classes of mood-altering drugs.

Target: The Female Consumer

Although they like to be thought of as public service institutions, the self-described ethical pharmaceutical manufacturers are among the most profit-minded industries in the world, and the most profitable pharmaceutical companies are those whose major sales are psychoactive drugs. It is estimated that this industry spends three or four times as much on advertising, sales, and promotion techniques as it does on research. In the case of mood-altering drugs, the promotional push has been particularly cost effective. Growth, both in production percentages and in gross profit per product, is greatest for those fortunate companies that have succeeded best in designing disease states — in enlarging the whole concept of illness — and thus designating the need for these broad-application, symptomatic "happiness" pills.

At a congressional hearing before the House Select Committee on Narcotics Abuse and Control in 1978, a representative of the Pharmaceutical Manufacturers Association (the lobbyists for the industry) was questioned by the chief counsel about the dismal, unattractive women seen repeatedly in medical journal ads. The unabashed response was:

> Illustrations in medical ads, as in all ads, are designed to attract the attention of the reader. They typically depict individuals whom the physician will relate to his own practice — people like those he's seen in his own office.

Let's look at how the pharmaceutical companies depict those people that *he* sees in *his* office. Using quasi-medical jargon to describe very real problems, the ads in medical journals aim to trigger responses in physicians' recognition of the stressful experiences of many of the women who populate their waiting rooms. Through this language, over the years, pharmaceutical companies have defined certain "diseases" as "environmental depression" and "empty-nest syndrome" and then come to the rescue with first one chemical cure, then another, and yet another. Many of the drugs with different patent names are, in fact, copycat drugs or combinations of drugs, all in the classification known as benzodiazepine, better known and loved by too many as Valium, Librium, Librax, Dalmane, and others. These are the second generation of the "mild" tranquilizers sired by the meprobamates Miltown and Equanil.

Typically, in the single, double, or four-page ads that fill the pages (and the coffers) of the medical journals, one-half to two-thirds of the layout is pictorial. The visual impact is heightened by a phrase connoting a diagnosis. To the busy professional reader, the female-patient message is clear, regardless of the compressed small type that fulfills Federal Food and Drug Administration (FDA) requirements for indications of use, problems, and drug composition.

Thus, under the headline EMPTY-NEST SYNDROME, a full-page picture allows us to look inside five unpeopled rooms in what was clearly once a busy home. The dining room is empty of all but furniture. The bedrooms, with toys still in place, make it clear that once there were children. The attic is filled with remnants of a lifetime passed and stored away. At the bottom of the page, sitting all alone in the living room, is an attractive, middle-aged woman. The companion page urges in large bold type: TRIAVIL FOR DEPRESSION WITH MODERATE ANXIETY. And in just a bit smaller type: "In Many Cases a Result of the 'Empty-Nest Syndrome.'" In the text, the ad describes the "midlife crisis" as a critical crossroad during which depression and anxiety are common. To treat it (only its symptoms, of course!), this coping compound will provide simultaneous antidepressant and tranquilizing therapy.

There are many physicians, it should be noted, who feel that such combination of drugs is irrational. Furthermore, experts in pharmacology urge physicians to be wary of providing tranquilizers to those who in fact may be suffering a truly medical depression — an illness caused by physiological imbalances — because such treatments could actually heighten the depression, not help it. Even the ad for Triavil notes at the very bottom of the page that "suicide is a possibility in any depressive illness. The patient should not have access to large quantities of the drug." It also says that anyone suspected of an overdose should quickly be hospitalized. Having shown this woman to be all alone, how specious it is to suggest quick treatment for an overdose. Who will see her in time?

Medical Advertising and the Elderly

In the August 1977 issue of the *Journal of the American Medical Association*, a grateful-looking elderly lady is pictured accepting a tablet from a clearly caring, young female nurse. In the center of this full-page ad are a few simple paragraphs under the headline TRANZENE HELPS YOU RELIEVE INSTITUTIONAL ANXIETY. The first paragraph describes "institutional anxiety" as distress related not only to health but to *the nursing home or the institution itself*. The second paragraph tells the doctor that the drug is efficacious and equivalent to the diazepams. This reference is designed to make prescribing more comfortable, since diazepams are part of a family of drugs that most general practitioners have learned to dispense freely to women of all ages. Finally, the doctor is told why this old therapy in a new name is more appropriate: It permits once-a-day dosage; it is easier to administer and costs less to provide, saving the institution staff many hours of dispensing medication (but depriving the patient of a few minutes of human contact).

Almost without exception, medical journal advertising designed to promote medication for the elderly depicts women almost surrealistically as shrinking, wizened little people, or as the unseen problem element in a tense family scene. The theme of the ads is that patients are troublesome and cause problems when they are awake, and are thus clearly less stress-producing if they are less aware, less active, asleep, or at any rate, controlled. These drugs are always suggested as management tools, sparing institutions or family members the inconvenience of the elderly female's sleepless nights or upsetting confusion. There is rarely even a cynical attempt to pretend that the patient's well-being is the primary reason to prescribe the medication.

The life crises go on, and no female is too young to be helped. The pharmaceutical company Pfizer advised doctors that Vistaril can reduce childhood anxieties. Accompanying the portrait of a tearful little girl are the words: "School, the Dark, Separation, Dental Visits, Monsters." On the next page the physician is urged to help when "the everyday anxieties of children sometimes get out of hand."

For the older (female) student, Librium may help her get "back on her feet" when "afflicted by a sense of lost identity in a strange environment, ... concerned over competition, apprehensive about national and world conditions, and confronted by the possible consequences of her 'new freedom' [which] may provoke acute feelings of insecurity."

Chemical solutions for other everyday human problems:

• "For anxiety that comes from not fitting in." Serentil.

• "You can't set her free. But you can help her feel less anxious. Beset by the seemingly insurmountable problems of raising a young family and confined to the home most of the time, her symptoms reflect a sense of inadequacy and isolation." Serax.

• "M A. (Fine Arts) ... P.T.A. (President-elect) ... with too little time to pursue a vocation for which she has spent many years in training ... a situation that may bespeak continuous frustration and stress." Valium.

Finally, Abbott Laboratories' "me too" tranquilizer, Tranxene, has been promoted in the form of a cynical ode to "what she doesn't know won't hurt her":

• "A different tranquilizer. Times change ... — A change of look ... is a physically distinctive change of therapy. It's very different in form and appearance from any other tranquilizer your patients have previously received or seen. —

Yet the same effectiveness . . . clinically equivalent to diazepam in treating anxiety."

Occasionally, disaffection with particular promotional devices has caused certain alterations or corrections in advertising, although changing very little in the prescribing habits of already captured doctors. Seduced by the industrial helpmates, doctors have unwittingly been reduced to the status of handmaidens to the new high priests of our medical culture — pills.

Senator Gaylord Nelson of Wisconsin, former Chairman of the Senate Subcommittee on Antitrust and Monopoly, who has been outspoken in his concern about the unhealthy practices of the drug industry, has said:

> The companies make claims through heavy promotional campaigns they know very well are not justified from a medical standpoint. They convince doctors to prescribe these drugs for purposes for which they shouldn't be prescribed. In my judgment, the present situation is intolerable. I do not believe that any doctor should base his drug prescribing on information received from advertising and promotion . . . The whole field of prescription and over-the-counter drug use is simply out of control. I think that the drug industry has outwitted, outspent, outinfluenced, pressured, successfully cajoled the medical profession, particularly the AMA, the Food and Drug Administration, the public, and the government.

The Role of a Pharmacist

There was a time when the neighborhood druggist was called "Doc." He knew everyone in the community and played an important, comforting role in health care. That local professional was respected for his concern and advice. He was reliable, available, and was the front-line intermediary between the physician and his customer. Now, the few pharmacists who own their establishments are mostly discount tradesmen or franchised dealers for distributors of house brands of packaged drugs. They manage a business, leaving others to deal with the public and the cash register. In most communities, chain-store outlets — primarily convenience one-stop shops — hire and fire their highly trained pharmacists in much the same way as they do other clerks. The major distinction is the placement of these specialists in an isolated, protected space, connected to humanity by a phone, with only occasional personal contact.

Just recently, waiting my turn at the cashier's line in such a market, I was witness to the following scene:

A clerk called over the loft barrier to the druggist: "Joe, that saleswoman from Sandoz (a manufacturer) wants to see you."

Locking the door behind him, the pharmacist emerged and greeted his visitor, who said, "I know you're busy and I promise not to keep you long. But you know I've just been working this territory for a few months and I need your help with some of our mutual clients. Okay?"

"Sure. No problem. How can I help?"

"Well, can you give me some idea which local docs are writing 'scrips'?"

"Well, Brown and Gordon are good. Barry, just fair . . ."

Looking at her clipboard, the saleswoman asked, "How about Thomas? Springer? Johnson?"

"Springer, yes. Thomas, poor, Johnson is getting better."

"How about my products? Who's writing? Young?"

"No, sorry, Young never does. Barry is coming on, but Healy is really big for you."

"None from Young? Whew, better do something about that. I've got my work cut out for me. You've really been a

big help. I'll be back in about a month, and by then you'll see
some changes. Meantime — think oral. And oh, this is for
you." The saleswoman handed him a small package, book
size.

He smiled and said, "That's really nice. Thanks a lot and
good luck." As the saleswoman left, the clerk and the druggist agreed, "She's cute and on the ball. She'll do fine."

Juxtapose that event with one other. Both happened within
one week, in the same place. Again, I was in the store. A
major news story had hit the nation. Dr. Peter Bourne, Special Assistant to the President for Health, had issued a questionable prescription for Quaaludes, a sedative-hypnotic tranquilizer. The networks and local media were all scurrying for
a different handle on the incident. A camera crew from a
nearby network affiliate was engaged in debate over company policy with the pharmacist. I overheard a cameraman
say, "But, sir, all we want to do is film the pills, or whatever
it is, so viewers can identify the stuff." The pharmacist was
adamant, insisting that "no pictures of any products can be
taken without approval from the main office."

The television crew spokesman tried to convince the druggist that their request was in the interest of providing good
graphic information, that they would limit their shots and
would not compromise security or the name of the store, and
that they would take into account any other logical consideration that might cause concern.

Nothing would do. The pharmacist insisted: "Ethics and
privacy rules are involved here, and it's my job to protect
them."

Incredulous, I wondered how this retail pharmacist could
interpret those lofty measures so differently for public information purposes than he did for the manufacturer's representatives.

A Detail Man's Story

I have, of course, no way of knowing whether that "on-the-ball" manufacturer's representative, with her list of neighborhood doctors and their inclinations to prescribe her company's products, will "do fine," as the pharmacist predicted. From time to time, though, I have met people in the business of promoting and selling "health" who have had to come to grips with their personal integrity and conscience. This story, told me by one disillusioned pharmaceutical detail man, is worth relating at some length:

> I was always interested in chemistry, even as a kid. I really wanted to do something to help people feel well and stay healthy. I couldn't go to medical school — the war got in the way, and I suppose a bunch of other things did as well. But I did graduate from college with a degree in chemistry. I had a driving wish to help, a degree to make it possible, and I was very ambitious. Becoming a salesman for a pharmaceutical manufacturer seemed a pretty good thing to do.
>
> I'm not sure whether everyone is naive, but I was — even about what drug companies' intentions really were. For the first several years, I really buried myself in all the papers and all the courses I could take, on the chemistry of the drugs I was promoting. I worked with a good bunch of guys, and I learned as quickly as I could from them until the cracks started to open up. I saw my own friends fall into them.
>
> The company pressure to sell more and more, especially tranquilizers, where they made their greatest profit, was tremendous. You get so caught up in the system. Your salary increases and bonuses depend on meeting sales figures, you've got a mortgage to meet and a family to take care of — all of these things are pretty distracting. For a while you really don't think about what you're selling so much as how much you're selling.
>
> There is so much fancy footwork. After a group of hearings before Senator [Edward] Kennedy's health subcommittee, we were no longer able to use words like "samples" or

sales "quotas." Mr. Clark, the company president went before the committee at the time they were describing free
samples as "payola" to doctors and pharmacists. Clark assured the Senators that *his company* did not give "samples"
and did not use "quotas." He did not say that our samples
are known as "clinical trial supplies" and "starter" packages!

In fact, all we had done was change the words. We were
probably sending out more free goods than we had ever
done when we called them "samples."

There is always somebody from the company negotiating
with the folks at the Food and Drug Administration. Every
so often they make a breakthrough. They convince somebody over there that our drug is safe for some other use
beyond the original purpose. As soon as they get clearance,
we have a new sales pitch to make. For a while, I used to
look forward to some new uses or new research, because
it would give me a chance to change my pitch to the same
group of doctors and pharmacists that I had to see over
and over and who had heard my old sales stuff about my
tranquilizers for a couple of years.

We had pretty good classes in ways to impress even old
clients with familiar drugs. Hell, half the time the doctors
didn't even realize how we maneuvered them into purchas-
ing more or prescribing more.

One of the sales tools we used is a question chart. It's
offered to doctors as a way to find out what they *don't*
need any more information about, regarding a particular
drug that our company really wants to sell more of. We
tell the doctors that we don't want to bother them by re-
peating information that they already know. We get them
to fill out this form, which tells us exactly how often they
use a particular drug, for what diagnosis, who they largely
give it to. Of course, the company's real purpose is to find
out where they *haven't* yet applied its use. They use this
information to shift advertising directions or in the next
discussion with the FDA.

Let me give you an example. Suppose Dr. A, thinking
he's going to be spared the same old sales pitch on the
usefulness of our tranquilizer, writes that he prescribes this
drug to a particular age group for just one or two syn-

dromes. When that pattern comes up in several regions, the company knows that it's time to shift gears. The next campaign, then, instead of focusing on anxiety for a particular middle-aged female group, might talk about muscle strain or stomach aches brought on by a family crisis or new-town stresses. Then we have new material.

When we started to find out something about the half-life of a drug, where it worked on the brain, and how long it would stay in the body even after a person had stopped taking the medication, some doctors were interested, but most I spoke to weren't. All they wanted to know was how much does it cost and are there any bad side effects. They really didn't care what happened to the whole body. Let's face it, if I referred to the hippocampus or the medulla and they didn't respond with interest, it wasn't going to help my sales or friendship with them to continue, so I just stopped. Sales were the bottom line for the company, and, of course, for me.

You get on to a terrible treadmill. It's something that I didn't understand for several years, that tricky business of trying to balance original ideals — "do something well and do some good" — against the backdrop of a design to only make money. I had a strong sense of being a professional, not a used car salesman or a life insurance salesman. The job pressure by division managers is pretty intense. You walk the fine edge of a double-edged sword. It's hard to live with yourself. If you have the responsibility of a wife and kids you know that you can get fired any time, or not get an increased salary, you're really stuck in the middle. The company benefits. One day you wonder about who is being hurt in all of this and decide that it's everyone — you, your family, your health, and everyone else you've done business with. And you wake up to what you've been doing all those years.

It hit me the day I was standing in a pharmacy which was one of my better outlets. I watched a dozen women get their prescriptions of one hundred tranquilizers each, and I knew in my heart-of-hearts that not all of those women needed one hundred tablets of tranquilizers. I had done my job too well.

I had to get out of it. So did many of my friends — the

ones who were still alive. But they are not alive to tell about it.

The company makes you sign all kinds of papers guarding them against the possibility of any of us talking publicly about the tactics used. Frankly, most of us are scared, and so what we know is not understood by people who need to know.

2

Valium for the Lump in Your Throat

"TELL ME about yourself."

Even as I heard myself saying the words, I wondered how many hundred times during the past six years I had asked or in some other way implied that same question. In how many settings had I listened for answers from the unending scores of women who had overcome drug addiction or counseled others?

How many national drug-abuse conferences had I attended at which federal bureaucrats established "official indices" and other references to establish that year's funding before disquieted but financially dependent health service workers and local administrators? With proper studentlike respect, I audited the paper presentations at polite scientific colloquia. Regardless of who the participants were, very little discussion in formal sessions dealt with living, breathing, and diverse people.

And I was troubled. Why was everyone so able to cast the human dilemma in such genderless generalizations? Why were the arguments more concerned with quasi-scientific premises — different from year to year and guru to guru? New evaluation "instruments" made it possible to manipulate survey data, depending on the incestuous idiom of the

assembled group. Where would real conversation take place?
Who would ask the question about the human exceptions to
the survey data?

For years, the special problems of people with different
skin color, different advantages socially, educationally, and
economically, and the issues of sexual preference and gender
consideration were largely ignored. Neat equations are not
easily drawn from too many variables. As an official of the
Food and Drug Administration once told me, "We tried to
include females in our test data on methadone during the
application period — but the damned hormone considerations just muddied up our need for quick results." Even now,
to some degree, those disruptive issues are relegated to rump
sessions, special caucuses, and anecdotal reviews. In effect,
they are outside the mainstream of social or scientific inquiry.

As the proverbial fly on the wall, I observed and analyzed
programs, professions, and profits, the better to understand
their separate and cumulative influences on people in pursuit of "the good things in life," including health.

In my growing awareness of the size and indiscriminate
reach of the drug problem among women, I vented my anger,
the result of my queries, in resentful articles, warning that
the female gender was becoming endangered. I wrote and
spoke to commissions and seminars, imploring those with
special interests to take off their blinders and, for the sake of
the future health of us all, to be inclusive and, in the spirit
of Abigail Adams, not to forget the ladies.

The Pharmaceutical Manufacturers Association newsletter
of July 31, 1978, quoted from my testimony before the House
Select Committee on Narcotics Abuse and Control, as follows:

> It is impossible to understand how, for so many years,
> right up to this date, the government has either ignored or

mishandled the substance abuse problem of over one-half of our country's population ... the incestuous relationship between industry and regulators ... wars between bureaucracies ..."

According to the newsletter, "Muriel Nellis, national project director of the Alliance of Regional Coalitions: Drugs, Alcohol and Women's Health, had a bad word for everyone — except women."

The Female Fix

But most of all I listened — to women, to their stories about themselves and about others who were important in their lives. I found no stereotypical female addict or addiction. But in that diverse, pluralistic universe, I recognized many common themes. I heard the subtle and apparent truths about our chemical culture — how its siren song may mesmerize any of us and that it threatens all of us. I learned that we share a most compelling circumstance: We all conduct our lives in female bodies, along historically parallel paths, in culturally private worlds. It is the essence of the "female fix."

Although each culture draws distinctions between appropriate male and female functions, women have always received mixed messages. Contrast, for example, the image of the stoic, pioneering woman, shouldering the enormous family and home responsibilities with the image of an unworldly, delicate-natured woman, subject to frequent "vapours and distempers." The combination results in a woman who, while performing her household duties with uncommon strength, requires protection and help for her inherent weaknesses, particularly emotional ones. To some degree, these culturally determined characteristics, our heritage, have become a self-fulfilling prophecy.

Troubling though it may be, there is compelling evidence that one of the factors in the propensity among women to resort to chemicals in coping with problems relates to frustrations encountered while trying to exemplify the contradictory images portrayed by tradition. The preference for legal nostrums may well be the result of a woman's sensitivity to social expectations, in fulfilling her "proper" role. Professionals who provide care and services act on presumed feelings and needs. The therapeutic marketplace has realized its most significant growth in those areas that best reflect traditional assumptions regarding the female condition.

In analyzing the stresses and vulnerabilities that are common denominators for women, making them susceptible to drug and alcohol dependency, I have learned that women who use drugs and alcohol are not a homogeneous group, but are young, old, rich, and poor, living in cities, suburbs, and rural areas. Each woman views her options from a different perspective. How we resolve our needs for strength, friends, or even escape is significant in determining whether, when, or what chemical dependency may develop. What coping alternatives are available? Which of these is most acceptable?

But despite the diversity of personal histories contemporary patterns of drug vulnerability are identifiable. Transitional times and events in the female experience appear to increase the likelihood for chemical dependency, for they call forth special needs that may produce emotional and physical discomfort. Inevitably, at these points, women are likely to require some kind of support. Troubled times and feelings are often subtle rather than apparent, but most common among the internalized, often unspoken feelings are those of loneliness, perceived isolation, and a lack of self-confidence, which may induce a sense of inferiority or even worthlessness.

I'd like to introduce you to Ann. When I met her she was thirty-one years old, the mother of Jenny, six years old, and Brian, eight. Ann's life — her values, her ambitions, her relationships — represents the basic profile of Middle America.

Ann married her high school sweetheart, and, to the pleasure of both families, they made their home nearby and soon began raising a family. Ann worked hard to please everyone around her. Never having considered herself especially pretty or bright, she was grateful for the security of familiar surroundings and traditional patterns.

When Brian was about three years old and Jenny was one, the serenity of Ann's life was threatened by limited funds and limitless demands. She began feeling weepy about almost anything. Her mother suggested that she didn't look well and that she ought to see the doctor before she might "give something to the children."

"I was accustomed to going to the doctor and taking his advice without question," Ann said, as she recounted her story.

> I'd been brought up to believe that the doctor is always right — that his advice was sound and in my best interest. Besides, I felt lucky that he took care of me.
>
> All he said was that I probably could use some iron and that Valium would take care of that lump-in-my-throat feeling. Just tense, that's all. And he was right. Once I started taking the medicine, I even slept better — for a while at least. I remember the day I discovered that the label said I could "take as needed." It was such a relief.

For almost a year, Ann punctuated each day with increasing doses of her "patience and fortitude" pills. When one pill didn't seem to make the needed difference, she took another. When still more didn't change how she felt, she thought she had "let the doctor down." Soon she began to feel frantic about everything.

> I know I should have told my doctor what I was feeling with those pills — but it just never crossed my mixed-up mind. I didn't even know how that drug could just pull a

reverse. I never talked to anyone about taking it, and no one warned me. But, boy, did I have my eyes opened. I finally realized I had a *real* problem. There I was — screaming at those two children who adored me, getting so worked up that I threw something at Jenny. Can you imagine? All they did were the things that all young children do — dropping things, spilling things, leaving toys around. Harmless kid stuff — and I went crazy enough to throw something? There I was taking Valium day and night to calm me down and I was hysterical. I became so frightened at almost hurting my baby that I called one of those "hot lines."

A trained counselor gained her confidence, assured her that her behavior was due to a serious drug reaction that was reversible with proper care and suggested some public and private facilities that could meet her need for help.

Ann's "habit" was sizable by that time (instead of the original fifteen milligrams, she was taking about sixty milligrams a day), and so her system required careful withdrawal from the drug. Had she simply stopped taking the tranquilizer, all at once, she could have gone into a mild seizure. "That call — and I don't know how I had the guts to make it — was a life line for us all."

You'd like Ann. After some counseling, reviewing her own priorities, she not only learned to ask questions, but how and why to require answers as well. She has a healthy, happy family, who have survived her need for self-discovery. Her aptitude test results confirmed that her previously unpolished doodling had artistic possibilities. She loves drawing and painting and, after a year of evening classes, became quite proficient at portraiture. When she isn't too busy, she accepts an occasional commission, locally, and she teaches part time. Even Ann likes Ann.

With just a few alterations, Ann's experience could have been Joan's or Dorothy Kilgallen's or Karen Ann Quinlan's. Joan played off her quiet pills against stimulants. After a couple of years, her erratic moods took such unpredictable swings that, when she lost her temper, she wasn't even aware of how severely she had punished her defiant child — who became one of the statistics of child abuse in 1976.

From Dorothy Kilgallen to Karen Ann Quinlan

During the 1950s and 1960s, few women in journalism enjoyed greater recognition in both print and television than Dorothy Kilgallen. Her coverage of the Sam Sheppard murder case for the *New York Journal-American* was, in the accepted fashion, sensational. Her grand entrances at posh New York parties produced an aura of success for the host and those who wanted to be mentioned in her columns. She was a *grande dame* of the popular program *What's My Line?* during its heyday. She lived in a socially glamorous and successful professional world in which casual drinking and daily use of a sleeping aid were commonplace. The coroner's report of Dorothy Kilgallen's death said she "died of the effects of a combination of alcohol and barbiturates, neither of which had been taken in excessive quantities."

Karen Ann was twenty-one years old. She had left her parents' home six months earlier and was sharing an apartment with a woman friend several miles away in New Jersey. In April 1975 she and a date went to a tavern for an informal birthday celebration in honor of a mutual friend. Her companion, Thomas French, said that they had had a couple of gin and tonic drinks earlier and that he had noticed that she had taken some pills. He claimed that they had only one more drink at the party, before leaving in his car. On the way home, she passed out, and he took her to the emergency room of the local hospital. She could not be revived. At the time, a doctor said that she appeared to have some metabolic imbalance, perhaps drug induced. Although her male friend characterized her as a self-destructive person, Karen Ann's roommate denied his statements, insisting that she was not a heavy drug user or drinker.

Although all of the events leading to Karen Ann Quinlan's collapse were never fully resolved, her tragedy eventually became the subject of national debate over parental rights to remove so-called life-sustaining equipment. The case went all the way to the New Jersey Supreme Court, where her parents' rights prevailed. Their Pyrrhic victory set legal precedent. Karen Ann doesn't know it, and we may never know more. She remains in a coma at this writing.

Reporting on the puzzling coma into which Karen Ann Quinlan lapsed, medical writer Maya Pines wrote that no more than a normally safe dosage of each of the following drugs had been ingested: Valium, Librium, quinine, aspirin, sedatives — and alcohol. (Chemical combinations draw their own deadly conclusions.)

Whatever the differences between these cases, at least two conclusions can be drawn from them. First, each one involved legally available drugs. Second, it is apparent that the burden and demands of survival may equally overwhelm those for whom life is "easy" as those for whom life is hard.

More than Biology

Are women physically and mentally less healthy than men? Even with increasingly aggravating factors — like cigarettes, alcohol, and increasing food and environment pollutants — by all accounts females live longer and, at each age, die at lower rates than males. Overwhelmingly, medical researchers report fewer female impairments due to digestive, circulatory, and infectious disorders. In fact, in that great survival-of-the-species game, women were dealt a biologically stronger hand.

Even if we concede that the female anatomy is more complicated because of the cycles and processes of its reproductive system (apparently bearing positive factors of physical benefits), the disproportionate number of women who have nonetheless become chemical cripples is not explained. Statistics alone don't define the dimensions of the human toll, the direct or indirect damage. One truth does emerge. The woman who has felt isolated with a secret "habit" is part of a growing constituency of potentially *accidental addicts.* More than just biology needs to be considered to understand this increasingly common destiny.

For many women, a deeply felt need for support produces a state of particular vulnerability. We aspire to see ourselves as we would have others see us — and the fear or reality of rejection becomes a heavy emotional taskmaster. Women, far more than men, will transform themselves — extend or withdraw — in search of approval, acceptance, or affection from those whose response will validate their growth.

Thoughts of private need might be entertained only secretly because they reflect personal — that is, "selfish" — concern. Often women squelch such needs to avoid the guilt. For many other women, the search for self and for personal substance is frustrated or thwarted by external forces. Furthermore, uncertain about the reliability of our instincts, particularly if they appear to collide with acceptable social patterns, we bandage our anxiety with such phrases as "learning to live with it," or "not letting it get me down." In some cases, such self-denial produces so much frustration that it is expressed in nonspecific but very real anger. Others seek safety, security, and confidentiality in the form of the advice and supervision of an authority figure. We seek legal, sanctioned comforts. We see doctors to be diagnosed, not judged. We present real symptoms, although they may disguise the underlying causes of discomfort. In many cases we are either unwilling or unable to identify carefully buried problems.

And we drink. It is acceptable. We drink to be sociable or attractive and to be less inhibited. We drink to find release and relief. We become hostages of legal drug and alcohol habits. We, who are the sisters, daughters, wives, and mothers of tradition, mask our moods for everyone else's comfort, to assure continuity and affirm our lives.

Chemical curtains have a way of parting, baring all our repressions in a new, strange form. From a mature perspective, Andrew recalls his confusion as a child:

> I expect I always wanted to be like my dad. He was a terrific, well-respected physician. But I remember being put in some miserable positions. I had to carry my mother to bed — up a very long flight of stairs — when she passed out from drinking too much. And I knew all the while that in between such bouts Dad would give her pills.
>
> It's strange — I now remember that my father was always in control of Mom's life, but I don't think he ever really seemed to know much else about her. She was a highly educated woman, but one who never got to show what she knew, at least not outside of the family. That must have been part of the problem.
>
> I can remember those times when Mom was "sick" and I had to take her home and put her to bed. They were awful times. That bright, gentle, good mother would get so crazed that she would strike out and really hurt me. Occasionally, afterward, I would try to tell her about what she had done just a day or night before. I even had bruises to show her. She would cry bitterly and, over and over, would deny remembering such events. In every situation, I felt terrible and comforted her. It was our game together, as though we were looking at someone else. We expressed pity for anyone who could harm a loved one.
>
> I now know that she never really translated that violent person into her own being. For a long time, I blocked out much of my home life and concentrated instead on a usually busy life during those growing up years. I'm not even certain which of us really ran away. I do know that in the process my poor mother was the one who had been, and remained, alone. Wherever she was, nobody noticed. We, all of us, removed ourselves. Now, sometimes my guilt exhausts me.

"It's a Girl"

In the middle of each adult exists a child who remembers what it was like to grow up. Sensations of well being or deprivation live on. At the core of the adult is the young life: early years of admonition or freedom, punishment or approval, happy relationships or ones restricted by rules governing interaction. Although we may not consciously relate our behavior to early events, spontaneous decisions and directions are colored by those prior influences. The judgments we make about ourselves and others are conditioned by the prologue of our personal journey through life. At every stage of our lives, much of what we lived and felt before is operational.

However, "It's a girl!" signals the beginning of a physical, emotional, and social life experience quite distinct from that of any male child. Recognition of the differences in our individual life experiences is no more important than a collective understanding of the parallel, often perilous, paths on which society and culture place us.

A very significant difference in the early conditioning of boys and girls is the degree to which boys have been urged to seek and take on challenges, in everything from competitive sports to exceeding the accomplishments of their fathers. Girls, on the other hand, have traditionally been guarded from, and admonished to avoid, "dangerous" — that is, risky — pursuits. They are generally taught to "play it safe" and not to venture into potentially jeopardizing, uncertain experiences. Unlike their brothers, girls are still rewarded for limiting their ambitions and curbing their instincts for adventure.

Along with this, there persists an anxious ethos regarding possible physical compromise — and subsequent societal punishment. One reason for this is that a girl's physical well being has implications for the future, for childbearing. An unblemished body and reputation were once viewed as critical to ensure that future.

Many of us had these protective messages. Although they were relayed in different ways, and with a variety of emphases, they have always been intended "for your own good." How many hours and years have women spent on analysts' couches, trying to overcome everything from sexual frigidity and fear of competition to the inability to make friends? These wounding phobias are often born of inhibiting reminders to "be careful, *they* only want one thing"; or, "Remember, people are always selfish — you can't trust them too much." How many of us dwell in lonely internal places of warnings?

The exceptions notwithstanding, most women lack the willingness to take risks. This characteristic is critical in determining the scope of our ambitions and can even predispose us to self-limiting expectations and subsequent feelings of being "trapped." When the possibilities of a positive return for an open, inquiring life are stifled, the opportunity for knowing one's own strengths is delayed, if not destroyed. We learn from experience. We each "own" our personal experiences. Each success, however small, produces a surer belief in one's innate or acquired ability. Taking chances is creative, positive, and, more than many other things, determines a way of life.

In some cases, living by the rules — by the values established by the institutions we accept — requires an unyielding compliance. Suppose you were Gloria, raised in a traditional Middle American family, one of three well-loved and well-disciplined children whose family, social activities, and religious life were all rooted in the same community. Respect for law and for the Orthodox Church was central to her upbringing, and it was completely appropriate for her to leave school in order to become a good wife. The rules that governed how, when, and why Gloria was to perform key daily tasks were historic verities, orderly and precise. The assumption that those truths were sufficient to resolve most crises was unquestioned.

In Gloria's case, a shift in time and tides brought about the need to make agonizing decisions. Her husband, Jerry, who had a promising new future in the town's new aerospace plant, suddenly found himself a casualty of the shift in political priorities and the subsequent budget cutbacks. But the cost of clothing and feeding their two growing sons was increasing each month; taxes had to be paid; the mortgage, car payments, and utility bills were outstanding; and now, three years after Bobby was born, she was pregnant.

The close-knit community in which Gloria and Jerry lived saw them as enjoying many blessings of the "good life." How they behaved, the decisions and actions they took, would undoubtedly be the subject of family and neighbors' judgments. Gloria knew the general attitudes of her own community — they had all pretty much adopted traditional values. In a single moment, these were all in jeopardy. For example, a productive citizen does not seek or accept handouts, especially welfare assistance, including food stamps; a trustworthy neighbor meets all financial obligations without pressure from creditors; a proper mother's place is in her home — she guards, instructs, and sets a good example for her children; and a God-fearing woman venerates prospective life, even more than her own — she may neither wish nor act in any way to harm it; a loving daughter and wife complains neither publicly nor privately — she maintains a nurturing, normal-as-possible environment and reinforces everyone's comfort by denying or dismissing even the appearance of problems.

When life was reasonably simple, it had been easy for Gloria to accept and live by the requirements imposed by family, church, and the social and business community. But where were the answers for her now? Where would she find the strength to question the appropriateness of abiding by all of those rules even if they produced no answers? From what separate source of courage could she draw on to begin to trust unorthodox survival instincts? Who could she really be angry at? And how could she not be angry, or at least frustrated? It's very hard to hold on to a sense of sufficiency or competence when one becomes so thoroughly dependent on outside forces and events that don't lend themselves to simple, personal intervention.

The disharmony that results from too many messages is implicit in Gloria's case. How could she, on the one hand, be concerned with the family's reputation for meeting debts and yet not be able to help her husband by trying to earn some money because, on the other hand, to be a proper mother she had to stay at home? How could she avoid detection of their humbled circumstances and still seek proper physical care for the prospective new child? With the admonition of her church, how could she avoid feeling guilty that she wished there were no new child in prospect?

Jerry determined that while his severance pay would cover most bills for a few weeks, there was no time to waste in finding new employment. He decided that a job would more likely be available quickly in the nearest large city, sixty-five miles from home. Gloria stayed behind, in charge of the holding pattern. Among other things, that included assuring her family that they "were just fine" and becoming unavailable to friends in order to avoid casual discussions of the situation. She waited, worried, punctuated her days and nights with aspirins for constant headaches, and troubled no one. ("There would be plenty of time to talk about this pregnancy, when I could do something about it.")

Within a month, Jerry found a job, at a reduced salary. Since he had to commute, Gloria had to manage without the car. Occasional and then frequent job demands made it necessary for Jerry to stay in the city. Increasingly, the customary drink before dinner became a solitary ritual. It quickly became Gloria's surrogate friend and make-it-through-the-night excuse. On one of those fuzzy nights, unable to sleep, she stumbled down a dark staircase and suffered a miscarriage. The crisis brought her husband and parents to her side with concern and assistance. Catering to her understandable debility, everyone came together to share the responsibilities of home, children, and chores — which earlier only she had borne.

Gloria burrowed into her secret self, burdened with unspoken guilt. When she left the hospital, she did so with a great many pills — some to ease her physical distress and others her overweight condition. Over a period of several months, she withdrew into acceptable, reclusive recuperation, where, privately, she also waited for certain punishment. It was she who really punished herself. Increasingly, her moods fluctuated between an almost frenzied need to do everything (thus appearing capable and worthy) and complete retreat from responsibility — into bottled sleep.

The night of Gloria's suicide attempt may have been the first time in her life that the rules were so openly thwarted.

Thereafter, Gloria made several other unsuccessful efforts to "end it all." Now she is hospitalized and under care, and her physicians continue to try to stabilize her emotional and physical upheavals with newer drugs and counselors. The children live with their grandparents; Jerry visits her religiously, every week; and the community continues to "understand" about her nervous breakdown after the "accident." For Gloria and Jerry everything has changed. Yet, for the community and its basic institutions, the rhythm of life is as it was. Good neighbors understand acceptable form and shy away from involvement in disturbing substance.

Freud defined depression as "anger turned inward." Many women like Gloria, who find themselves unable to determine practical, personal paths and who are afraid to risk unsettling the secure rhythms established by the institutional systems in their lives, are diagnosed as suffering from "anxiety with secondary depression." They retreat from the community world into a private one where liquid or solid drugs provide therapeutic relief, while time passes. Removed from the circumstances that raise doubts, they are insulated from the judgment of those who may decide their actions are improper.

In recent years, many group discussions with women have focused on the two-sided coins that make up the complexity of the human condition. For example, the need to belong may, alternatively, promote the fear of rejection. For every easy measure of what one "should do" there is an implied "should not."

The Critical Stages

On top of the cultural characteristics that predispose females to accepting supporting roles, there are certain critical events and stages that tend to heighten feelings of need and therefore increase vulnerability to bottled and capsuled comfort. If H. G. Wells was correct in warning that "more and more, history is a race between education and catastrophe," then a review of these troubling times may produce life-saving signposts.

The difficulty of the adolescent years for females has been well documented throughout several generations. At that juncture in life, girls are confronted for the first time with taking individual actions that result in acceptance or rejection from several groups or individuals in their lives. Wherever I listen to women discussing their problems, more times than not they refer to their adolescence. Their present concerns and dilemmas are the outgrowth of early rules and expectations, rewards or defeats, and they are couched in recollections of that period beginning at about twelve years of age.

Joanie was an introverted, overweight child. She fantasized her social life and expressed it in writing, beginning at twelve years of age. By fourteen, in 1965, she had authored six "of my own books," most of which were loving encounters with teenage music idols. But, yearning for participation and acceptance in real terms, she stopped "tearing hardcovers off my mother's valuable books to use as covers for my own creations" and agreed to see a psychiatrist. She was counseled to take diet pills, wear dresses, and "look cute," and to join with others her age (who were occasionally smoking pot). Her solitary creative inclinations were considered antisocial and were therefore discouraged.

By the time she was eighteen, Joanie's circle of friends had grown and the social rituals included Methadrine and Demerol. But she didn't like herself any more than her parents did. A year later, she applied to the local county vocational rehabilitation program for financial aid to attend a community college. She recalls how demeaned she felt by the interviewing psychologist. In order to qualify for this assistance program she had to detail her history of drug deviance and agree that she was "a sick person," that her tendency to wear black "was proof that I was seriously depressed." No one ever cared about her repressed instincts to be creative and her desire to be a slim, attractive person. She took the county's largesse — one year's tuition — but felt humiliated and uncertain of her right to redemption, and lived up to the expectation that she was antisocial.

At age twenty, cut adrift from her family, Joanie decided to come to terms with herself. She began writing again and stopped using drugs; she moved away from old friends and from everything that had made her captive to a limited, self-destructive image. The first year was excruciatingly lonely, except for her job in a bookstore. She read and learned on her own and earned her way back to school, on her own terms.

She had, however, lost so much of her childhood that six years later, she was still looking for self-definitions that were not borrowed. Today, she continues to search her diaries for clues to her future potential. In her letter to me, she noted that her "guilt still shows," and she recounts,

> I was, I think, a very screwed-up kid, always overweight and being reminded of it. Only recently have I had real hope for even learning to like myself. I think my past drug use was a symptom of angers and frustrations I didn't even know were there.

During this past generation in particular, the teenage years have been times of increased conflict and crisis. In the struggle for maturity in an adult world that emphasizes that young women should be beautiful but affords them insubstantial functions, the pressures to be popular, to adapt to changing social mores, are intense. The youthful population has been larger, more mobile, and financially and socially more independent than in earlier generations. The nuclear family has grown increasingly less stable. Young women, who are expected to behave responsibly, by virtue of greater peer-group involvement are more likely to define appropriate behavior through the limited experiences of their youthful friends. If the explosion of communication and other technologies has resulted in traumatic pressures on adults, who find decision making increasingly difficult, imagine what uncertainties this fast-paced world creates for young women. The social pressure to assert one's individuality in a highly mobile world of change is coupled with incessant examples of acquisitiveness, might-makes-right, and instant gratification, which in sum produce complex choices and great uncertainty. Now the opportunity as well as the pressure to drink and to experiment with lifestyles and drugs have made these things factors of daily life for the young. As for mixed messages, how effective are adult admonitions against the use of drugs by adolescents when these same adults are of a generation committed to medical drug therapies?

Recent studies in California, monitored over an eight-year period, have shown that young women are increasingly using alcohol and cigarettes at rates exceeding those of young men. Moreover, the pattern appears to be consistently true throughout the country. Many people believe that it foreshadows a similar trend in drug behavior.

Teenage females are more sexually active at much younger ages than previous generations. These young women have also been in much more frequent contact with health-care providers. Twelve-year-old girls are given tranquilizers to cope with their new social experiences and are prescribed opiate-derived pain killers, such as Percodan, to relieve menstrual discomfort.

Young women of the sixties and those of the seventies are fully aware of the overindulgence of mature people in the use of alcohol and prescribed legal drugs. They grew up with stocked medicine cabinets, from which many of them received their first introduction to drugs that were supposedly safer than those on the streets.

Barbara recollects that, as "a child of the sixties," she had experimented with many of the street drugs of those rebellious times. However, her serious addiction — to pain killers — began in her early twenties, when she recycled an attention-getting back ailment that she had first experienced at thirteen.

Barbara's life had continued to be tumultuous in her twenties, as she searched for the approval of parents, who had been embarrassed by her friends and earlier lifestyle. Her father was a prominent member of the community in which they lived, and Barbara used his relationships with local physicians to secure what became a three-years' supply of pain-killing drugs. She now recognizes that even today her greatest temptation to return to the use of those drugs is to blot out the pain of never having succeeded in developing a relationship with her father. "That drug made me feel warm — like being loved."

The external worlds of adult women and all teenagers bear some striking similarities. The contributions that both groups expect to make to the institutional mainstream of society are restricted by cultural, legal, and hierarchical stipulations. The youthful years are characterized by inhibited function and undervaluation, as are the lives of women in general. Likewise, both women and young people live in a tense, temporary space as they try to adapt to life-role demands.

Growing numbers of teenage girls today are runaways, victims of domestic violence, refugees from unloving homes where one or both parents may have abused alcohol or drugs. Nancy's history of drug use is inextricably bound up with her family life and particularly with her mother.

Nancy's Story

When Nancy was in high school, her mother was in her late thirties. Nancy and her three sisters were aware of their father's increased absences from home and knew that their mother was certain that her husband was interested in another woman. In addition, the anxiety over the uncertainty of available money to pay bills or buy clothes was constant.

> My mother and her friends started going to the doctor to get diet pills. They were overweight. First she started taking them about three times a day. Every so often she had to get weighed by the doctor and get some new prescriptions. My mother is a terrific cook. She used to eat a lot. First I

noticed that she stopped eating, and I asked her about it. She'd just say that the medicine curbed her appetite. It made her smoke a lot more, too. Pretty soon she started acting real jittery and nervous. All kinds of things would make her wild; things that came up at school that made her angry would provoke her into hitting us. She'd grab one of us, shake us a lot. She started acting real crazy.

It is worth interrupting Nancy's case history here to explain the immediate and long-term effects of diet pills. Originally, stimulant drugs were considered to be of great benefit, with very little risk of serious side effects. We have since come to understand that this group of drugs is particularly troublesome. Most prescription problems involve amphetamines and related compounds whose actions arouse the central nervous system and thus physical and mental activity. Drugs like Preludin, prescribed to women for weight reduction, are characteristic of these drugs. Although they do depress the appetite centers of the brain for a short duration, the regimen of continued therapy by many "diet doctors" is lengthy and therefore contrary to both safe and effective use.

Too often, particularly in the lives of women confronted by long days, disturbed nights, and many demands, these drugs become the mainstay of functioning. Even a standard prescribed dose may produce an unusual level of wakefulness and reduced fatigue. These drugs excite respiration, heartbeat, and blood pressure, causing frenetic activity and jittery restlessness. After continued use and heavy dosage, mental depression and exhaustion are common. True to this profile, Nancy's mother was openly anxious, angry, and tired — almost simultaneously.

Since amphetamines act for several hours and need to be taken increasingly often to be effective, high dosage levels are reached quickly. Many women need either a minor tranquilizer or eventually a sedative in order to accommodate the body's need for the rest it has been denied.

Nancy is certain that her mother's effort to lose weight and shape up had to do with her wanting to be more attractive to her wandering husband as well as trying to improve herself sufficiently to show him that she was not wholly dependent on his taking notice of her.

> After she started taking the pills and losing weight, she decided to "do something with her life." For a while she started taking courses to be a nurse's aide. Something happened to that; I don't know what. She lost all interest after a while and dropped it.
>
> She had a full-time job taking care of four of us. She started getting more and more hyper. She couldn't handle anything. She kept screaming and yelling. It wasn't like her at all. Even her language started getting terrible. She started saying a lot of stuff I knew she didn't mean, but it really hurt our feelings.

In addition, their father had a history of drinking too much and then striking their mother. The absence of stability in the parents' relationship was confusing to the girls when they were younger. Why, they wondered, would their parents hurt each other in the name of loving each other? But even when, as adolescents, they offered sympathy to their bruised mother (whose personality had by then been altered by her drug use), they could not be sure of her response to them.

> We would reach out and tell her how sorry we were for her pain and then feel stupid. She would cry, "I don't need you here." And then she'd get so nasty, so downright nasty. She thought we were interfering, but we were just trying to help.

Going home became a last resort for all of the girls. The erratic, painful atmosphere, devoid of positive family relationships, made it a place to avoid. Companionship and lessons in values and conflict solving were better found at school or at anyone else's house. The one message that came across to the girls from their mother, inadvertently, was that one could "leave home" emotionally and seek remedy for personal problems in the chemical change offered by pills. Their first experience with altering their own dreadful environment was through trying the uppers and downers in their mother's medicine chest. "I guess we all had to run away quickly and in as many ways as we could."

Nancy and her sisters proceeded to experiment with different lifestyles and drugs of all kinds. Apparently it was easy for their behavior to go unnoticed, since both parents were caught up in their own chemical and emotional traps.

> I didn't have any nice clothes, I never went to a prom. I couldn't afford a gown. No one asked me, "What do you want to be when you grow up?" There was no point to it. Trying to find some fun each day — making the most of it was all that mattered. I really messed up my life. Skipping school, bad crowds, and at eighteen — married. All of us picked the wrong people. I got married mostly because my father was so against it. I wasn't married very long. I hated it so much. My sisters did the same thing and they were no better off. I wasted so much time. All of us got so involved with the wrong things — all alike.

After surviving bad marriages and critical involvement with drugs and alcohol, Nancy and her sisters, at different stages, undid their scarring pasts. Nancy exercised self-determination. She helped herself and nursed one sister through a "cold turkey" drying out. Pregnancy caused another girl to seek medical care. The third completed a halfway-house program of treatment. Now each is in pursuit of a more realistic life.

Although it is true that any one of the many negative influences in Nancy's life might have been significantly disruptive, it is worth noting that, at a critical stage of adolescent growth, drugs and drinking were the escape behaviors learned at home. Nancy and her sisters were not aware until many years later what great effect that had had in reproducing both the vacuum and the violence they had sought to leave.

The flood of contemporary self-help books that examine family patterns or relationships with parents has brought into the mainstream the theories of such experts as Freud, Erik Erikson, and Robert Coles. We can now readily learn how many of us spend a good bit of our lives trying to resolve our conflicts, either by rejecting our childhood relationships to our parents, or by seeking to confirm those early messages that dictate all our subsequent behavior.

Only recently, however, has it been acknowledged that drugs and alcohol are among the primary alternatives to coping with or working out those internal problems. Studies indicate that adolescents from families whose parents use alcohol regularly or depend on over-the-counter or prescribed medications (particularly those that effect a change in mood) are three to seven times as likely to use both legal and illegal drugs and alcohol themselves than are children who do not receive the subliminal message that comfort is found in a bottle or a package.

3

The Unprepared Mother

MANY YOUNG WOMEN barely out of adolescence embark prematurely on married lives, either because they feel the need to run away or to pursue the continuity of early marriage traditions. The ability to fulfill solemn vows of "forever," along with the responsibilities they bring, is put to especially difficult tests in today's complex, uncertain society.

Very young women are too soon confronted by the realities of their limited experience, income, and skills. Their storybook fantasies are replaced by less glamorous impulses for survival in often dismal conditions. Whether they believed, or wanted to believe, in "happily ever after," for too many the myth is shattered too soon. The kind of emotional discontent that weaves throughout the unfulfilled lives of these young women leads them to seek some level of sufficiency. In some cases they may begin to drink, alone or with their young, hard-working husbands. Other young women, feeling unfulfilled, become pregnant.

Baby: Reality versus Fantasy

The "need" for a child is often not so much a conscious choice as it is the absence of one. Or it may be a subconscious desire to confirm oneself in the one way available to all young women capable of reproduction, regardless of their particular abilities or their social and economic circumstances. Pregnancy is a time for care and attention, if not from one's own family or husband, then surely from a professional who must, in a regular fashion, attend to the physical comfort and the needs of the potential mother and the unborn child. For many young women the prospect of motherhood offers a promise, the promise of being loved unreservedly, almost as one receives affection from any small pet. And a baby is one's very own pet — and responsibility.

When a young woman is pregnant, whether she wishes to be or not, new decisions or burdens emerge. The more youthful the prospective mother, the more she will inevitably need support, advice, attention, and affection. Depending upon her support network — where she gets advice, how she is comforted, if at all — her sense of self and her instincts for survival will either be strengthened or shaken. Even assuming the best possible circumstances — namely, a husband who is enthusiastic about the prospective first child, the birth of a healthy child, and her own young health intact — that first year and a half of complete submission of self to the unremitting needs of a new life often makes such emotional as well as physical demands on the young mother that her self-confidence is tested in every conceivable way. Around her, the larger world goes on, and so must she — in one way or another.

A well-known pediatrician once told me that "more times than I like to think about, I have to resist the temptation to accede to a young mother's request to 'please do something to calm this baby down,' because the mother looks so terrible and needs some sleep."

Another said, "I think I spend more time counseling young mothers who are riddled with guilt, because they have felt so much animosity toward the demanding baby. I've told them no one else has a better right. It's okay. You can say it. You can feel it. No one will punish you. Stop punishing yourself." And, "I give more prescriptions to the young mothers for their nerves than for their children's illnesses."

Easy or difficult, single or married, motherhood is a stage of life for which women are almost universally unprepared. That is true even if emotional instinct is strong. Because we must, throughout a child's first years, rely so often on our untrained responses to parenting, self-doubt and uncertainty are frequent, troublesome visitors. Then, just about the time a woman feels comfortable and secure in established patterns of mothering, her children's full-time dependency on her is transferred to other people.

The Children Grow Up

Although some young women busy themselves in auxiliary roles that relate specifically to the growth of their children's community interests, for others it is the first time in many years when there is enough quiet time for personal reflection. Perhaps it is the first chance a woman has to review her satisfactions or dissatisfactions. It isn't that there aren't many other things that can be done after the yellow school bus leaves. The real issue is the personal sense of deprivation, the loss of unique purpose. One woman told me,

> Once I got over the tears I shed at the first leaving of that school bus — you know, a little bit anxious about whether or not anyone would love Bobby as much as I knew he needed love, that sort of thing — I was overjoyed at the prospect of having some time to myself, to read a little bit, which is a luxury I had to relegate to tired evenings before. Pretty soon that wore off. Oh, I belonged to the PTA, and I helped make the costumes for the class plays. But one day it occurred to me that when I had been the one to do

everything, I had also gone to bed a lot happier, even if I was more tired at night.

I guess the best part of being a mother is not so much what you do or have to do, but that only you can do it. Somehow you get to know that you're very important and that what you're doing is the best in all the world for your own children.

Little by little, experts, professionals, even friends become just as important in the life of your children, and you have to surrender some of that unique relationship, that personal sharing and giving — and receiving — that was your very own. And I became a little lonely. I missed feeling special. It was as if someone had just jilted or replaced me. I wasn't sure what my new full-time mission should be.

A strange thing began to happen. Tom started questioning me — a little testily — about what I had done all day. He really made me feel guilty. And so I started looking for things to do, in order to be able to report to him at night. I know he was under pressure. Expenses were growing, he was ambitious and wanted to move ahead, for all of us. So I tried to be understanding. I kept the house just the way he wanted it and tried to please everybody more of the time. But I shared in less of their lives every day and had fewer of those moments that made me feel special and filled empty places.

It all began for her so innocuously. Twice a week, after helping to collect and sell at the local hospital's white elephant shop, a long, wet drink with coworkers was welcome and deserved. An occasional headache or backache was common, and just the right thing was handy in someone's purse. It was like finding a good recipe, and since she didn't like to wait for another's offering, she purchased the ingredients for use as needed. The lonely time between fund-raising events and other neighborly good work efforts was made less troublesome by more frequent use of time and pain chasers. Two years of scheming to beat the clock, to keep up appearances, and stay calm turned into sleepless nights, tearful days, and a determination to be done with this artificial life.

Her young husband told me, in an authentic state of shock,

> I just didn't believe it. I really thought we had a good marriage. I really thought she was happy. I was working my tail off and she was hitting the bottle. I never saw it. And the pills — my God, I had no idea about the pills. Now the doctor tells me that she went through hell trying to undo a really heavy habit alone. And it turns out that she blames me. She says if I had really cared about her, I would have noticed. You could have knocked me over with a ten-foot pole. I came home and found her gone and the note said it was all my fault and she wants a divorce. She says she needs to go back and find "the girl and the promise I lost somewhere." I thought I knew her. Somewhere, when I wasn't looking, another woman came into my life — I just never noticed. How could I have known?

Perhaps knowing would have made all the difference. He wasn't looking carefully, or he would have noticed that his sparrow had lost a wing. Instead she found chemical crutches, which then put her in jeopardy. In search of survival, she sought her own strengths — by herself. It's altogether likely that a different woman had, in fact, emerged.

If the instinct for giving grows stronger but the need for that support and service is lessened, a disquieting imbalance sets in. The consequences are varied. Some women become angry. Others, embarrassed at their needfulness, fearful of letting it show, may seek new outlets, with or without regard for old standards of safety.

In whatever way this dilemma of diminished importance is handled initially — by ignoring it, submerging it, or filling time — it is, at best, a transitory coping technique, not a solution. Unless the sense of personal abandonment or loss is recognized, other patterns are likely to form and may take uncertain turns or become crises. Dr. Estelle Ramey, an endocrinologist who is a professor at Georgetown University, described one visible form. She commented on the "disease of free-flowing boredom in so many physicians' offices any day of any week. Why it's almost a club. They meet regularly and brag about how many medications and how many doctors are 'taking care of' their particular ailments and headaches."

The divorce statistics clearly suggest the tension or vacuum that characterize the classic seven- to ten-year itch. A good part of that has to do with a breakdown in communications, a breakdown of the sensitive dialogue necessary to alert two people to each other's needs, whether or not verbally expressed.

Both men and women have got to confront some basic facts. Men suffer stress, both physical and emotional, during the years of maturing and parenting. Their stresses are almost universally related to jobs, careers, economic advancements, and other tangible dilemmas. However, many of the stresses suffered by women involve that combat zone of self-definition: overcoming internal guilt over wanting to be somehow untraditional, being torn between their own dreams and the expectations of the world around them. Their behaviors are measured against time and chores, and in neither case is there constancy or certain reward. In many ways, the longer a woman seeks to be identified with someone else's achievements and growth, the more certainly those very things will deprive her of self-definition.

Four Mothers, Formerly Married

Four women came to meet with me. The differences in their ages represented generational spans of approximately twenty years. They had very different lives except that they had all been married, had children (in one case, five), were now unmarried, and could reflect on their separate histories, all of which were nearly short-circuited by drugs or alcohol. During our lengthy discussion of the ways in which each had embarked on a chemical regimen, one area of agreement emerged. Whether prior to or during the use of drugs, each woman was aware of feeling an emotional exhaustion that was related in some way to her long-time need to respond to the expectations of others. One expressed it this way:

> There's something that happens without warning. I don't even know when I started living constantly for other people. And everywhere, that's the only attitude that gets reinforced. I would say to my son, "Pick up your room. I have friends coming over. It has to be neat." What was really going through my mind is, "I'm a good mother and good mothers take care of the house. Everyone who sees that will know, will be satisfied, will be happy."
>
> I tried so hard to be perfect that it grew painful. I had stiff neck muscles, became edgy, and then sought relief in pills. First a little, then all the time. And all the while there was this commercial on television to keep me stupid. Now it makes me so angry, I want to smash the set. It's the one that equates good and bad mothers with doing clothes in a particular way. Every time I see it I'm reminded of how I exhausted myself for what turns out to be nothing more than a hard sell — a television commercial image.

Another woman elaborated,

> It took me years to realize that the resentment and anger I suppressed was really fear — fear of facing myself. I was afraid that I'd find a weak, selfish person. We can talk theory until the cows come home, but it all comes back to how you feel about yourself. Then you have to be willing to say "I've had it," recognizing that whatever way you were coping wasn't the answer and give it up. Try something else. The only way to find peace is to find faith in yourself. Then it's all much simpler.

Diane talked about how difficult it can be to create one's own strong self-image when all of one's training is geared to submitting to the needs of others.

How do you find the courage to question what you've been fed since day one? I knew my place, and it wasn't leader.

I've got to tell you a story. I was married very young. My husband and I both worked, saving for the future and a family. One day I was on duty in the operating room. The details don't matter, but a terrible mistake was made and I went into shock.

I had a complete breakdown and had to be put into a hospital. I got all kinds of treatment — shock treatments and the drugs. I had carloads of drugs from three different psychiatrists, and I could renew the prescriptions, which I did, for years. When I was released from the hospital — and I was scared to death to face my family, whom I had embarrassed with my mental illness — everyone wanted to make me feel "normal."

To show their confidence and to celebrate my return, I was given a huge glass of whiskey and everyone toasted me. I can remember the terrific feeling of relief. The drink numbed me into calm. But I resumed my life, went to work, took care of my young family, and turned to the bottle whenever the pressure got to be too great. Only my husband knew; I was careful never to drink in public. But I couldn't get through a day without it. To keep him from objecting, I went along with his decision to be in charge of my supply. Every day when I left my job I filled a half-hour with chores, giving him time to get home first and fill my jelly jar with a big Manhattan. Like a playful puppy, I would beg him for the drink he kept hidden. It was a cruel game, but I didn't care; I needed it so much.

Through it all I managed to raise my children. They too were married young and left home within two years of each other. I began daydreaming about how I might start saving my salary for things I had never done, like travel, but everyone else's plans became my chores. Free time became babysitting. My husband bought a campsite for family holidays, but I was expected to shop and cook and continue to do more of the same chores I did at home.

My husband wouldn't hear my dreams, but soon they were all I cared about. There had to be more to my life or there would be no reason to go on. I had done everything for everyone else; now I wanted it for me. I left my husband after twenty-nine years, took trips alone, and drank until there was no place to go.

When I went to AA, it wasn't to stop drinking. It was to find some understanding, some kinship, some peace. And that's what I found. But it wasn't easy to unsnarl the turmoil of a lifetime and to find and trust myself. For the first time I've got my own act together.

The afternoon ended on a note of total agreement that I've heard from others as well as Chris, who said,

Dealing honestly with yourself and others takes a lot of energy. Whatever it comes from — and anger will do — you've got to have a selfish strength to dig out all the things that really trouble you and dump them. Share them, understand them, surrender them — I don't care what words are used — just let go of the things that won't let you go. You've got to recognize what's garbage and come out from under the weight of it. Without that load, there's energy to change, to feel alive.

4

Working Women

THE WORLD TODAY is, as we know, more open to greater freedom and opportunities for women. In the professions, in the job market, in competitive sports, gender is less an obstacle to ambition than it used to be. But the metamorphosis is slow and viewed by many with a wary eye. Some tradition-bound fundamentalists openly disdain women's chances, claiming that such change seriously threatens the order of the future. It is a complex matter — this business of having our certitudes shaken, of no longer being able to count on things being predictable. As with any alteration, this stress, too, produces emotional responses and casualties.

Single women at any age find themselves segregated from those who have married. Whether their status represents a choice to remain unattached or is a transition period, these women may be viewed as threats to insecure, housebound women or to fragile marriages. One woman expressed consternation over her recent rejection by a former friend. She discovered that her newly married chum was barely interested in hearing about any successful accomplishments that were once a mutual ambition. She told me:

> It's so hard to understand. Once we all dreamed together, talked about success. But if one of us breaks out, takes those

steps, makes it, all bets are off. No one makes the way easy, not even those women. Instead, the battle begins in earnest. I suppose that none of us is really free from society's lessons.

Whether or not this woman could fully appreciate the fears or emotional adaptations behind her friend's apparent distance, she had been unkindly cast off. In this case, as in many others, faith in the ongoing reliability of friendship becomes tainted by suspicion, an obvious step on the path to defensive isolation.

The Social Ghetto

Curious about this barrier to expanding support networks between women, I've discussed this shadowy "unwelcome" sign that separates them into insulated social ghettos. Many young wives admit to having pulled away from their former, single friends or knowingly having resisted the companionship of women who remain uncoupled. Some have told me that they "really hadn't given it much thought." Others rationalize and offer the easy "we just don't have much in common." One, who tried to be introspective but became uncomfortable, pondered,

> My guilt comes to mind. The women's movement has only scratched the surface of female America. We don't know why, but some of us at home feel anger at the few who have "made it" as professionals. If we try to verbalize it, we may be told that we're crazy, that we "have a problem." It's troublesome. Frankly, I've got enough to worry about without that.

Yet, in times of crisis, we all need others. Support and understanding are not arbitrarily divided into categories of "married" or "single." Nor is despair or loneliness. Just as the working world is providing greater numbers of women common experience, both single and married women are having to cope with job pressures. For one thing, "equal opportunity for women" is in many ways still tentative. Women who choose to pursue a career face a world where their contributions are considered less valuable and are less well compensated than those of their male colleagues. And there are other "dues" exacted.

Sandy's Story

Sandy's first twenty-two years of life were insulated from brutality by a successful and loving family who encouraged her ambitions and were able to provide her with a first-class education at a prestigious Eastern school for women. When she graduated, she insisted on making her own way in New York.

Culturally accomplished, energetic, and remarkably good-looking, Sandy recalled that her first few months of job hunting were marked chiefly by the culture shock of living in a large, competitive city and by the number of men she met who tried to take her to bed. Although she found the attention flattering at first ("attractiveness seemed a positive attribute when the interview lines were long"), soon it became a distracting, pride-bruising maneuver. With no job in sight, her rigid determination to find her own way was getting shaky as her money supply ran low. "I couldn't let my parents know any of it. They would have insisted that I give it up and come home. I would have felt like a failure."

She grew to hate the game playing, whether in the job hunt or on the phone with her family, and her discomfort caused insomnia. Her frustration and uncertainty often reduced her to tears when she was alone. A little brandy helped a lot.

Finally, her perseverance paid off. Sandy was hired by a midtown advertising agency to be an assistant to a senior account executive. It was an acceptable position for gaining some specific skills and experience and the future held promise. Her boss was businesslike, considerate — and married. Sandy was glad for the opportunity to work on an important project with Jack, even if it meant staying late to help meet a business deadline. In short, Sandy felt secure — until the sexual advances began.

At first Jack's flirtations were barely perceptible, but then the pressure began in earnest. Accidental touches turned to deliberate embraces. His whispered comments about "how sexy" she looked became "Let's go somewhere else tonight . . . There's something else to look at besides ads." The more Sandy politely dodged, the more persistent was Jack's pursuit. The only thing that helped the tension headaches at night was Valium. Sandy began to feel defensive. She was certain that Jack's increasing, intimate overtures were being noticed by others in the office. A martini at lunch calmed her anxiety, temporarily. But the whispers and glances of her fellow workers continued. Jack's demands did too.

Finally, after her department transfer request was denied, Sandy was instructed to accompany Jack to a two-day meeting in Boston. She flatly turned down the obvious setup. Jack sent her a memo in which his warning was clear. Using such veiled phrases as "need for more extended commitment to company interests" and "must improve cooperative attitude," he promised dismissal if her refusals continued.

The prospect of losing her job was terrifying. That fear collided with angry disgust at the notion of having to prostitute herself in order to work. She ached all over and left the office "sick." She bought some vodka and, during the next couple of days in bed, tried to blot out thinking at all. It was worth the hangover. The next month was a hectic period for the company and, blessedly, for executive business. Oppressive episodes with Jack were kept to a minimum and Sandy had established a relief ritual. With martinis at lunch, several more at dinner, and tranquilizers "as needed" for sleep, her dry heaves lessened. She could eat dinner and keep it down.

But the day of reckoning with her sexual blackmailer came. Sandy remembers returning to her apartment after work to confront her world of limited options.

> I thought of my job — how hard it was to find it, how much it meant to keep it. I remembered the months of need, of pretending to my parents, of sheer exhaustion from trying. Was I to blame for being exploited? Had I invited propositions? Would there be a Jack wherever I worked? Was I anything more than just a sex object? I couldn't find the answers, so I kept drinking. I lay down on the couch. My heart was pounding so hard, I decided to take some pills. I just don't remember another moment of that night. I woke in a strange bed, in a hospital room. My body felt like a truck had run over it. My head was bursting. A doctor came in and told me how lucky it was that a neighbor had noticed that my apartment door was unlocked and partially open. If the ambulance hadn't come quickly and if my stomach hadn't been pumped, I would have died.

Sandy left New York and went home to safety. She was fortunate. Other young women don't have that choice.

The Working Mother

Today's married, working woman does more than overtime. Often she is expected to adapt her job responsibilities to her "proper" roles of loving wife, gracious hostess, good mother, and community volunteer. Whatever her role or responsibility, on the job she must be twice as competent, learn to fit in like one of the boys, and demonstrate her comfort with accepted rituals such as travel, corporate parties, and late-hour deadlines. She may learn to drink like a man in order to perform like a superwoman.

At thirty-four, Sally returned to work when her two chil-

dren began to attend elementary school. She felt pretty lucky
— her husband was moving up in his law firm and now she
would finally have an opportunity to put her own hard-won
education to the test by working at a job in her field. Of
course it was going to be a little difficult to get the kids off
to school, put herself together, manage the unreliable bus
schedules and get to work by 8:45 in the morning. But she
could handle it — she would just start her day a little earlier.
It was a long day, and it soon became apparent that she'd
have to be more alert for those 3:00 creative planning sessions. Four cups of coffee didn't seem to do it. A friend at
work suggested that what she needed was this "wonderful
little pill" and offered her some.

It worked. Sally went to her friend's doctor and he prescribed the same amphetamine for Sally because she, too,
was "tired" — and besides, it might help her lose some
weight. All that extra energy even made the late afternoon
marketing, the stop at the cleaners, and cleaning-up after
dinner less difficult. The only problem was that she couldn't
shut her mind or body off in order to go to sleep.

After a couple of weeks of sleepless nights, she needed
more of those pep pills to keep her awake during the day
to meet the demands of her job. And now her heart was
pounding too fast.

Back to the doctor. He gave her a new prescription, this
time for a "mild" sedative / tranquilizer. Now she could regulate her waking and sleeping patterns. And she was certain
they were safe because, aside from the prescribed three-times-
a-day dosage, the label read, "Take as needed."

Nobody told her that her highs and lows would become sharper and that she'd start taking one or the other
of those pills to counteract problems caused by them. She
began the day in a fog — that is, until she took a pep pill.
That made her irritable and impatient with her coworkers,

and rather than throw a fit, she took a drink at lunch.

One evening, after Sally and her husband returned from a festive champagne dinner in celebration of their anniversary, Sally took her nightly sleeping pill. She soon felt dizzy. Her face was numb and she had trouble focusing. Before she could force sound through her sluggish lips, she fell to the floor, unconscious. Her husband grabbed the phone and called for an ambulance. The rescue-service operator assured him that help was coming, told him to check her breathing and look for signs of bleeding, and asked if he had any knowledge of what might have caused her collapse. Since there were no obvious clues, he was instructed to gather any medicines his wife might have been taking, including patent remedies, to give to the medics on arrival. Sally's breathing was light and very slow. Her hands were cold and she looked extremely pale. Scavenging through the medicine cabinet and the nightstand drawer, her husband found empty pill containers. From her fallen purse others had been scattered on the floor. As soon as the rescue squad arrived and saw the bottles, they radioed ahead so that the emergency-room team would be prepared to take correct resuscitative action.

It was only at the hospital that Sally fully understood the torturous ritual she had been putting her body through. She had survived what could have been a lethal combination. (She might have become an apparent-suicide statistic.) Fortunately, the tests taken of her vital functions were good and there was no sign of heart arrhythmia or other damage from the amphetamines. Now all she had to do was assure her frightened husband that she had only meant to spare him the clinical details of how she had been coping, that she had intended to use those medicines only while she was "adjusting," that she wanted him to know she was not a drug addict. At least she didn't think so.

Single Mothers

More young women than ever before are being counted in the census as heads of their families — that is to say, they have dependent children for whom they are the sole support. Each year nearly one million teenagers become pregnant — thirty thousand of them are under fifteen years of age. Increasingly, these very young women are deciding to have their babies and to keep them. When we add to the number of unmarried mothers the growing number of divorced mothers, we are confronted by a large population of women who must maintain a home and perform at least two jobs, one of which entails the enormous responsibilities of motherhood.

Single mothers share a common problem with those who are divorced and left with young children: they are alone with economic burdens. The census figures indicate that more than nine million families are headed by women. Many of them work at low-paying jobs, maintain homes for their children, are constantly beset by money problems, and live in fear of illness or some other crisis that cannot be met by either their single incomes or limited other support resources. Maintaining the very necessities of life is such an overwhelming responsibility that there is often very little time for either friends or recreation.

Pat has been divorced for three years. Her former husband is remarried and relocated across the country. At the time of their divorce, Pat assumed sole custody and financial responsibility for their daughter. Mary Ellen is in the first grade, learning to count; her mother is thirty-three, a typist, counting-down to emotional exhaustion. She's a candidate for help. I heard the symptoms:

> Oh, what I'd give for just some time — to finish a book, to hear some music, to be free of that too-many-chores-for-one-day feeling. I feel so responsible for so much — and for

so long. Oh, how I hate to feel like a martyr. It makes me angry — which makes me feel guilty. My God, it's a "snow day" — no school, no one to help. Where does the time and money go? I'm always worried and tired. Sometimes I wonder if that child knows . . . or cares.

Cathy, a waitress, was paying for her own night classes at business school when she became pregnant. She moved from her aunt's home (where she had lived since she was orphaned, at six), far enough away to avoid any hostile judgment. Now she is reluctantly questioning her decision. At ten in the morning her sighs are heavy with alcohol, as she seeks help from a counselor at the social services department.

It's not that I don't love my daughter. It's just that — well, sometimes there's just so much, it crowds my mind and body. The dull, unending chores; the new experiences I can't risk; the opportunities I miss, or worse, don't notice; everything mixed up with backaches, headaches, colds, and dentist bills. Days are full of crying, shopping, inoculations and schedules. And then there's the unscheduled chicken pox. I can't do it all, that's all — at least not all at once.

The problems of the single female who is the head of her family are exacerbated should that woman be economically deprived and fall into the dehumanized cracks of our institutionalized systems of welfare and other labeled largesse. On the one hand, the medical care and counseling available may provide excessive supplies of calming drugs (that cut down on the patient load and returnees at public health institutions) and at the other end of the spectrum, should she develop a "habit" — either solid or liquid — she may risk being declared an unfit mother for seeking assistance and have her children removed "in their best interest."

Both Pat and Cathy made certain choices. Each woman was purposeful and courageous, and each intended to be a responsible mother and productive citizen. But their environments were different, and so, too, were their ways of trying to remedy similar problems. Pat was no stranger to her community. She soon discovered that among her office friends and within her neighborhood there were others, even in two-parent families, who needed a helping network. She shared in the effort and benefited from new friends and freedoms.

Cathy's road was less smooth. The case worker who discussed her four-year file with me explained that the child welfare department had had no choice but to place her child in temporary foster care homes on three separate occasions when Cathy was unemployed and during her hospitalization. Her expenditure of welfare funds was scrutinized, her ability to provide a proper place to raise her child was reviewed, but no one questioned what else she swallowed down with her pride, unseen. She had been fired from one job after another for arriving late, missing days at work, or not performing with full vigor. Was it depression, exhaustion, sedative hangover? According to the review file, it was any or all of those, but no one could reconstruct the order in which they occurred. However, Cathy decided to rebuild her priorities and regain her daughter, and the welfare board is now ready to return the child. Cathy believes that her health is only in jeopardy when her self-respect depends on the intervention of a distrusting system.

5

Her Husband's Career

EVEN GEOGRAPHY imposes peculiar stresses on women. I learned a lot about that when I served as coordinator of the first nationwide assessment of conditions that affect the health of women, with special focus on drug and alcohol problems. The following passage is from my report to the Department of Health, Education, and Welfare:

> In much of Alaska, winters are long and bleak. Life is frequently hard, especially for women. Many are newcomers who have followed husband and job but have no extended family or friends, no place to turn in adversity. Jobs are hard to find, wife battering is common, and the divorce rate is 52 percent higher than the national average. It should not be surprising that the use of alcohol and drugs is high or that the "at risk group for abuse" (among women) includes all but the very young and the very old. Nor should it be surprising that... drug users and alcoholics are bored and lonely people having trouble adapting to the severe climate, to the drastic cultural changes...

And, I might have added, to the absoluteness of their depending for comfort on everything external to themselves.

But it is not only in Alaska that women have problems, much as that environment, harsh and demanding in extraordinary ways, does intensify such problems. My report to

HEW reviewed the plight of rural women in general: "In a rural community, few opportunities are available to women who wish to expand the realm of their existence and little exists in terms of cultural activities, continuing education, or an opportunity for professional status." Such limitations, omnipresent in the lives of these women, often spell misery. Alcohol or other sedatives are logical companions, masking the dullness of life and the absence of human interaction.

Also implicit in the lives of rural women is their economic dependence on the man of the house and their almost total isolation from family and friends. But there are parallel stresses in the lives of urban women who live in crowded ghettos. In many instances, their experiences of enforced isolation and lack of opportunity produce the same deprivations that confront women in Alaska and the rural communities of our country. Additional barriers compound that deprivation, including economic and material limitations, cultural constraints, and often an inability to speak English. Whatever causes isolation in the lives of women, whether cultural or linguistic alienation or distance from others, a limited horizon causes the same response: turning inward.

One of my colleagues in Utah did a study which showed that 69 percent of women over the age of thirty-four who were not employed outside the home and who were members in good standing of the Mormon Church use minor tranquilizers. By the time they reach forty-five or fifty, these women are considered a major risk population for addiction. And these are facts about a population that places great emphasis on sustaining the nuclear family and its future, a population in which women carry out the most traditional responsibilities of the female role.

Excessive drug and alcohol dependence also appears to be the travel mate to dutiful wives who become the casualties of their husbands' careers. Constant transience, with its repeated uprooting, results in acute anxiety and subsequent depression. The problem is particularly noticeable among the wives of military men and foreign service and corporate professionals. These moves are at least disruptive of continuity and are often traumatic for women who must always begin again to find new friends and make a place for themselves and their families in each new community.

Carolyn's Story

Carolyn has just celebrated her forty-eighth birthday. She belongs to a self-help group whose members have all experienced a personal crisis with drugs. Even now, two years after her last pill or drink, she explores her past in a continuing effort to understand the pathways of her own vulnerability. Her desire is great, her ability to savor the future, uneasy.

Until it became distorted by drugs, Carolyn lived a demanding but satisfying life. When she married Jim, he was already considered executive material by a top-forty corporation. She loved being his helpmate and hostess. Having grown up in a military family, Carolyn understood and responded well to a structured, hierarchical lifestyle. Her transition to a corporate existence was comfortable. Aside from having the expected, minor problems, Jim and Carolyn and their three children flourished.

When Carolyn was thirty-six, there came a year of crisis. Within a three-month period, her only sister was widowed and then suffered a stroke. Carolyn's two boys and her sister's son, whom she was tending during his mother's recuperation, came down with the flu. Jim's business-connected social obligations increased, while Carolyn's stamina was low, and conflicting priorities became the subject of argument and tension. Accusations led to recrimination and silenced anger. Tension took its toll, and Carolyn, untrained for such disorganization, sought to establish control.

She consulted one doctor and learned that she suffered from a spastic colon. Another doctor ministered to her painful neck. Both "treatments" worked; both were tranquilizers (one with codeine) and were depressant. Carolyn slept so much that she wasn't bothered by Jim's absences. She tried to attend to major duties properly but found that she had increasingly less patience and more confusion. At dinner parties she was more pleasant if drinks were served before and after. She listened and smiled a great deal and only spoke when she had to. Any occasion provided a reason for either a drink or a pill.

In talking to Carolyn later, I asked her to free-associate her recollections of just one traumatic day during her "run." "Can you remember what was on your mind?" She could. It was just after they had moved to a new city. It was the fourth move in Jim's career. The timing was difficult, moving teenagers in the middle of a school year, before Christmas. The company had found a house for them. She would manage. In less than a month Jim wanted to invite his new boss and his wife to a holiday dinner.

> I never thought I'd make it. I worried to death about whether the house was ready to entertain the Johnsons. At the same time, I had to bring extra pressure on the kids to make themselves scarce, keep the noise and music down — in general, to make a good impression. I knew Jim was counting on me. I was worried about everything. Was the new butcher truthful when he assured me that the roast would be tender? Had I bought enough? (I knew I spent too much.) Would the stove work or ruin my timing? Should I have hired someone to serve dinner? Will the Johnsons like me — enough to invite us back, help us to make friends easily?
>
> There was no end to the troubling questions, and my head began that familiar steady pounding. Somewhere in the midst of tending to the chores I knew by heart, I mixed a shaker of martinis and one of Manhattans and chilled them. I recall one especially uneasy moment. Just before

Jim was due home, I stood before the refrigerator door, reaching for "a small one, just to relax," and I couldn't recall whether it would be my third or fifth that day.

One morning Jim caught Carolyn fixing her "breakfast milkshake" — before she added the vanilla and cinnamon to the cream-covered Scotch. He tried to grab it from her. She went into a raging panic; she needed it so much. The pitcher fell to the floor, and Carolyn after it in shaking sobs.

Jim soothed Carolyn briefly and then, while she was applying cold water to her face as he had urged, he phoned a private treatment facility. Then he explained to her that he knew about this resortlike medical retreat, only ninety miles away. In the guarded world of corporate executives and professionals, breakdowns, whatever the cause or route, are treated with elegant discretion. The health farm that he called had been a rehabilitation setting for several of his colleagues. Some had suffered from nervous exhaustion, others from alcohol or drugs.

Once assured that Jim was fully aware of her problem and wanted to help, Carolyn let his good judgment take charge. He avoided making any specific reference to alcoholism. He spoke about the strain on her nerves and health and convinced her that a good rest and a thorough physical examination would help whatever condition was causing her trouble. He urged her to think of the couple of months ahead as an indulgence, a long-deserved pampering. (In fact, that's how he referred to her sabbatical at his office.) He helped her pack a suitcase and poured a "toast"; then they drove ninety miles "acting normal."

Because of her long, dual addiction, complete withdrawal treatment was more complicated and slower than anticipated. Even after leaving the farm three months later, Carolyn remained under regular medical care for recurring bouts of tremors, insomnia, and occasional disorientation. Constant testing had shown her endocrine system to be imbalanced; there was also liver damage. Continued memory-lapses and sudden bursts of rage have led to tests for sus-pected brain dysfunction or other problems of the central nervous system. Uncertain of the degree of impairment or the cause of initial trauma, her doctors try both drug and other therapies, alternatively and with restraint. Although Carolyn counts the morning when Jim stayed home from the office to take her to the health farm as her rebirthday, her health bears the scars of old habits and a second-gener-ation of disease symptoms.

The stress of constantly having to prove yourself anew, while at the same time trying to pursue a normal daily life, attend to necessary chores, and maintain the appearance of sociable calm for everyone else's sake, requires extraordinary effort. At the very least, both physical and emotional fatigue are very real prospects. The use of psychoactive drugs even-tually transforms what was intended as a Band-Aid into a tourniquet.

Families of Public Men

One of the better-kept secrets of public life is the extent to which the dependent family members of men in politics represent a large army of the walking wounded. The woman and her children are often denied the presence of the man of the house, yet their behavior in the outside world must always be careful and contained, since it potentially reflects on the reputation and career possibilities of that man.

Demands on a political wife to live up to an image are often in great conflict with the reality of her daily existence. To be an active asset requires constant availability for polit-ical and social events — great mobility. But, in order fully to attend to the needs of dependent children — within the constraints of a limited salary — a woman must necessarily restrict such activity.

The children of politicians must seek peer acceptance and experiential growth in a public space bordered by adult rules of comportment. In order to meet the various demands of this kind of life, these wives and children share little time together. However, they share a common vulnerability to mood-altering intoxicants.

Betty is a training specialist for a large, county drug-treatment system in Florida. She conferred with a teacher in the Cape Canaveral area about the drug problems among her students. Many are the children of space-age professionals, astronauts, and government officials. The teacher described these youngsters as having "disaffiliation" in common. She reported that they would gather in groups on the beaches to smoke pot and pop pills, "staying out of the way." She wondered,

> What can be done to give those kids something or someone to belong to? They have little or no connection to the technical world of their fathers, who are either in outer space or engaged in preparations for such flights. Their mothers are busy trying to handle a coupled life while bereft of husband companionship. They are unable to share in any significant work; they only function to enhance their husband's image and, thus, advance his career. Each family member has a special cocoon.

The often lonely worlds of the family members of public figures is fraught with veiled emotional turmoil.

The Congressman's Wife

Rita always knew her husband would run for Congress one day. Bob was a popular insurance executive and had been very successful. They had a handsome home in the Midwestern city where she was born, many friends, and an enviable marriage. Rita had a degree in interior design, but her plans to start a small business were interrupted when the local head of their political party persuaded Bob to run for Congress. Rita recalls the whirlwind campaigning:

> My hands got sore, my legs were weary, and I thought my smile would forever be frozen in place. I never knew that people belonged to so many clubs. After a while, I lost track of days and nights. It all became a blur of tomato juice, creamed-something, canned grapefruit sections, and coffee, coffee, coffee. At every stop, a new introduction — the same thing with some local inside color. "The pretty lady," "his good little woman," "one of our own," "helpmate," "better half," and even "special in her own right."

The simulated adulation, the frantic activity, the sheer repetition of waiting on the sidelines and smiling, all began to get to Rita. Bob assured her that it would be over soon, "when we move to Washington," a trip she secretly dreaded.

The beginning of Bob's congressional career marked the beginning of the end of their marriage. Rita tried to be a good sport. She flew back and forth to Washington until she found an affordable apartment, not too far from Capitol Hill. At first, Rita accompanied Bob to all the dinners, parties, and political gatherings that, as a new congressman, he was expected to attend. She used her decorating talents to make their home attractive and warm. And she hated it. She had no friends, she didn't know the community — except that it was unsafe at night — and shopping for everything was a chore. Bob's schedule was erratic. Dinner together became a sometime thing, postponed regularly by excuses: "I'll be a little late — I've got to stop by at Congressman So-and-So's party at six, then just a brief handshake or two at the Press Club."

Rita was unaccustomed to a social life primarily motivated by photo opportunities. She would occasionally drop by at Bob's office, but she always felt she was in the way. Her sense of uselessness grew as she observed her husband becoming more and more self-important and preoccupied with congressional business. She recalled:

> The little wife who played such an important role on the local scene felt more like a matronly dowager among the bevy of young women on the Hill. All those secretaries — seeking and giving approval, attention — all of them "on the inside" of my husband's most important activities. I handled my jealousy very badly. I became increasingly unavailable for his stupid parties; made fun of the long-legged popsicles in his office; and accused him of believing the myth that his press officer had created.

Rita succeeded in driving her husband further away — away from the derision at home that was in sharp contrast to the adulation and admiration he received everywhere else. His disinclination to spend time with her served to reinforce Rita's certainty that there was another woman, or other women. It fueled her resentment; she tried to drown that resentment with liquor.

Rita and Bob agreed that she probably should go home for a therapeutic visit. "Besides, I needed a checkup, and I didn't trust any of those strange doctors." Rita never told her doctor that she had started to drink. He had known her long enough to see that her nerves were frayed and apt to keep her awake at night. He supplied her with sedatives. He told her to stay put awhile and get some rest.

After a couple of weeks, Rita returned to Washington. Almost at once she could feel her jaw locking with tension. Now there were occasional gossip column references to Bob's being seen in the company of some attractive woman or another. She recalls,

> I couldn't eat. I was a nervous wreck. Like a damn fool, I fortified myself with alcohol and confronted him in his office. I was shaking all over, holding back the tears when I accused him of abandoning me and threatened to make him pay for it.

It was a particularly violent rage in which accusations flew both ways. Bob accused her of not caring about his career, of acting like a spoiled adolescent, not grown up enough to live in the real world of adults who matter. At the height of the battle, Rita blacked out. It was a traumatic event for both of them.

The next morning Rita took herself to a nearby Virginia physician who would keep her confidence and calm her nerves. She told me, "Librium was the one way to keep my hands from trembling without drinking, which obviously made me lose control." She decided that she wanted to exercise control of her life. She did not hate Bob, nor did she want to harm his career. She also did not want to share it any longer. They came to a civilized understanding. They would be publicly supportive of each other. Rita would return to their district in the Midwest and make that the base for her interior design business enterprise. When she came to Washington for major political events, they would share the Washington apartment. Similarly, when constituent business brought him to the district, he would stay at their local residence with her. They would each try to keep their private lives and needs as removed from public scrutiny as possible. And so their separate survival contract was struck. Only occasionally did the cracks show — and then in very limited circles. Recently a friend told me about a dinner party in Washington where he spent time with Bob and Rita:

> She wasn't drinking at all. She watched all of the rest of us drink before dinner and never touched a drop. Yet, when I tried to talk with her privately, I had the feeling she was off in space somewhere. It was strange. She was simply not with it.

From time to time, Bob received a brotherly piece of advice from colleagues. When on foreign trips or other official visits out of Washington, he was known to drink too much. Less charitable remarks began to be made:

> The damn fool embarrassed the hell out of all of us. He drinks too much, forgets to pay the tab, and sometimes he's an absolute lecher with women. The hell of it is, we have to protect him — make excuses for him — in order to protect ourselves.

Although Rita's and Bob's lives follow this pattern even now, it is a fragile blueprint, susceptible to crisis. Their individual and mutual future comfort is dependent on maintaining a controlled facade; their weaknesses are solitarily addressed with alcohol or pills.

This is not an uncommon political scenario. Depending on how much is really known about Rita and Bob or their relationship, Washington insiders either envy, admire, or scorn this political couple's solution.

The need to be circumspect has often meant that the dependents of men in public life, in business or the military, have sought help outside the view of the political, military, or industrial complex. This is beginning to change. These institutions are now dealing more openly with family problems and other behavioral crises.

Just six years ago, the public hospitals, clinics, and treatment centers in Hawaii were complaining that they had the burden of caring for the enormous military dependent populations with drug and alcohol problems. I am told that now the military hospitals are seeing these problems too. A young doctor at Tripler Hospital, an Army medical base in Honolulu confided:

> Half the time the waiting rooms here are filled with the saddest bunch of not fully grown-up mothers and their kids, whose heads are in a mess. They're so damn lonely out here and they haven't even become whole people. The

child-abuse problem is tremendous, and the violence within families is worse among adults.

As you go out, look at the battered women and bruises on any of them, including their kids. I'm here to take care of those physical problems — their pains. I can't do too much about the booze or the pain that doesn't show. Sometimes I think they come here just so that I'll give them something to bury all the rest. It's terribly sad. At least if they come here we can keep a check on how much of anything they're getting from us. I'm very careful about limiting how much of any drug I give them for any type of pain.

"Measuring Up"

The pressures to belong, to be good, to measure up, are positive motivations for many people. However, when that pressure is too great, too demanding, too unrewarding, some disruptive results are likely. That is particularly true if the strength of self is in question. It is also true if there are constant, uncertain goals that have to be met. Then the person's activity may become frantic, anxious, and lend itself to compulsive behavior and a constant mood of insecurity. This underlying current is often seen among not fully grown children who are forced by circumstance, environment, or choice to live and behave as adults or to function in an adult world too soon. It is also true among homemakers who have never come to terms with that undefined girl who, first known as "Sally's daughter," became "Bill's wife," then "Amy's mother," and who may then suddenly be confronted by transitions that further reduce her self-definition. The strength to accept losses in life — even predictable ones — is critically diminished if one lacks a personal, separate identity.

Alice came from an upper-class, socially conscious Eastern family whose only expectation of her was that she be "proper." The one experience in her youth that she recalls as a moment of self-assurance was her debutante ball, where she had the long-awaited first drink that dissolved her awkwardness and insecurity. She left college to marry her first ardent suitor, quickly had three children, and then her first divorce. After that, she began years of "knee walking" through life.

With her three small children, Alice moved to a quietly elegant resort community, where she drank to forget her loneliness.

> I tried to do all the right things, but I never could quite fit into it. The more I drank, the less I was troubled. I had the children to raise. Everything was difficult, filled with anxiety. I was depressed.

The psychiatrist Alice went to see convinced her to take a harder look at her drinking habits, then promptly prescribed tranquilizers to wean her from alcohol. For the next six and a half years she was on "this merry-go-round of pills. I took pep pills, diet pills, uppers, downers — everything. I went to more than one doctor, got a different variety from each." She was hospitalized several times for taking too many kinds of drugs, but her psychiatrist continued to help her try to find herself during that period.

> For some reason he felt that taking amphetamines was an optimistic sign. It showed that I was interested in being part of the active world. He disapproved of the depressants; they were a sign of detachment, removal from reality.

Finally Alice convinced herself that all of her problems would clear up if she gave up alcohol, and so she went to Alcoholics Anonymous. Her experience in this group gave her a great many things, including new relationships. One was with a successfully sober, mature man who, unlike her father, noticed that she was pretty and admired her talents. He married her; but within a year they separated.

That destroyed me, it really did. I was certain I had failed him, too. It took years for me to realize that it was a bad marriage — built of weak material — and it never could have worked. But I suffered so. I had tried to make it work. My judgment was at stake. Doing and being right were on the line.

Frightened and unsure, feeling diminished in the eyes of the community and degraded by failure, Alice ran away again, to a new city. She needed to succeed — desperately now — for herself, for her apathetic parents, and uninterested brothers, and for her skeptical children. To assure her good figure and positive attitude, she began increasing her intake of stimulants. She found a job as a salesperson but was frightened all the time. She took sleeping pills every night. Each day seemed just another reminder of her reduced status in life. She was living in a small apartment, "feeling left out and worried about letting everyone down."

I started having greater difficulty getting to work regularly. My income started to suffer, too. Christmas was coming and I was terribly worried about giving the children a good holiday.

I'm not sure whether it was perfectionism, pills, or the terror of another failure which drove me so hard. I had an overwhelming sense of having so much to do and an abiding fear of not being able to do it. I remember that as the worst Christmas of my life, and yet I remember very little of it. I felt exhausted as I took the bus home from work that evening. All the way, I took pills to pick me up. I kept thinking about the stockings I had to fill, the turkey that needed stuffing, and all that I wanted to do to assure a good Christmas. What I actually did was only told to me later, much later.

Her children went out to dinner that night with their teenage friends. When they returned, they found her in a frenzy, "stuffing the turkey all over the kitchen — absolutely out of control." Then she passed out. After waiting at the hospital to find out whether their mother would survive after having her stomach pumped and other emergency care, Alice's family went home. They put the trappings of Christmas away and didn't want to see their mother again.

After yet another round of remorse, pain, and trying too hard to improve her situation with pills, Alice decided to admit herself to the hospital for "cold turkey" detoxification.

> By that time, I was willing to do anything. I had done everything else so badly. I knew what I was in for. And I was right. I never felt so sick in my life but I was through taking pills against people forever.

For the past eight years, Alice has been sober, free from all mood-changing drugs. (The only exceptions were the pain medications given to her after several operations for heart malfunctions.) She has devoted herself to two major pursuits. One of them is the slow but progressive rebuilding of a relationship with her children. They have finally grown to believe her promises to remain drug free, just as she for the first time understands their earlier terror-filled turning away. With equal dedication, she works with public and private groups that provide help to addicted women.

Alice has not remarried, but not because she is unwilling or fearful. She is open to all positive possibilities and no longer lives with forebodings of disaster.

> I remember the first day I awakened to the fact that I had succeeded — after a lifetime history of failure. I came to the realization that I had not suddenly been struck well and good in that instant. It had been possible all along. For too long I had perceived each trauma as enormous. I had no sense of proportion. But now I have broken the idea of my personal failure. And although I may not succeed at everything in the future — the "worst" might happen — but it happened before. I now know I can cope.

The prospect or actuality of separation or divorce, whether it happens by design or comes as a surprise, produces great anxiety. Regardless of the circumstances, there is always a period of self-doubt. "Was it my fault?" "Could I have done something to prevent it?" "Am I unattractive, unworthy, lacking in wisdom?" "What will those who know me think of me?" And, finally, "What will happen next and can I trust my judgment ever again?" All of those introspective questions don't even begin to address other critical considerations: children, food, housing, life alone. Doing, being, anticipating unknowns — all produce symptoms. Someone or something is turned to, no matter how stifled the cry for help.

6

The Older Woman

AGING IS LACED with the myths of unspoken terrors. Often menopause signals the beginning of decline, in every form. Too often this threatening "change of life" coincides with the separation from now-grown children who had been the certain touchstone with youth and productivity. Where once a few peaceful hours alone were welcome, endless time to oneself becomes unending loneliness. Many middle-aged women spend too much time waiting to be invited into someone else's schedule, either their husband's career or their children's activities. Hours must be filled. Ladies' luncheons and shopping tours are diversions but not important. This empty routine reinforces negative self-esteem. Some of these problems can be masked with a chemical comforter . . . or several. Some of the least suspect may be villainous.

Hysterectomies and Other Assaults

Having recovered from extensive surgery and two weeks of heavy withdrawal from Premarin, an estrogen mixture, which I had taken for thirteen years, I feel that hormones should be classified with other drugs given to women by doctors to "calm" them during their "troubled age." All are dangerous and habit forming.

My college daughter knew more than my gynecologist.

She said I should not be taking hormones, but when I asked
my doctor he said that without a uterus and cervix I needn't
worry. "The hormones make you feel better and you won't
have hot flashes!"

Now I have blood clots and a dysrhythmic heart and an
experience in the hospital that was almost like death.

Receiving this letter caused one to recall earlier research
and the continuing debate over these drugs, prescribed for
questionable "benefit" to women. Are they addictive? Like
tranquilizers, they are given freely to females of all ages and
for a host of broad purposes. Young women by the millions
take them for birth control; a generation ago pregnant
women took another form to prevent miscarriage (and now
learn that they produced children with potentially serious
problems). Like the woman who wrote to me, thousands
more take some form of hormone-replacement therapy after
hysterectomies or the onset of menopause. Is this woman's
case exceptional? Probably not. Generally speaking, if the
body makes a relatively undramatic adjustment to a new
agent, it then accommodates that agent's presence and actions. The agent may effect changes, noticeable or not, and
it may precipitate an altered condition that requires other
chemical adjustment. This pattern is true of most chemical
regimens. Certainly, drugs that are derived from substances
said by the manufacturer to be involved in psychological
and emotional aspects of feminine behavior, drugs that affect
the master gland control of hormones, are likely change-
agents. As do other popular medications, these have as many
defenders to extol their virtues as they do opponents who
are troubled by known and suspected risks. The better-
known dangers of these drugs — phlebitis, increased blood
pressure, blood clots, and certain tumor enlargements — constitute the general issues of debate over their use. Less discussed are significant associations with migraine headaches,
depression, nervousness, irritability, malaise, and fatigue —

all symptoms that are disturbingly, insidiously like the warnings about addictive, psychoactive drugs.

Physical and emotional assaults regularly traumatize contemporary women, regardless of age. Whether the crisis results from a criminal act of rape or from wife-battering (a gray legal area, subject to state law), it is a violent insult to normalcy. A similar sense of invasion accompanies major female surgical procedures — mastectomies and hysterectomies. However, beyond this, the victim or patient is then faced with society's judgment that aberrations of any sort are repulsive — a threat to order and function, societal or individual. As a result, instances of assault or rape often remain unidentified because of the victim's shame and fear that, by virtue of her actions or inactions, her injury might be judged as deliberate, self-induced, or avoidable. It is the same vicious stigma that paralyzes many women who have become unintentional addicts.

Only recently has some serious study been given to the disabilities that women suffer after such experiences. There is mounting evidence that women who have concealed earlier violent encounters — in the streets, in their homes, or in operating rooms — frequently fall prey to long-term psychoactive drug use.

A team of researchers at Yale Medical School were funded by the National Institute of Mental Health to investigate the response of doctors to victims of domestic violence. Their 1979 study revealed that emergency room personnel seldom identified these women's injuries as the result of battering. The danger of ignoring that primary problem is aggravated by the fact that doctors prescribe tranquilizing or pain medication to one out of four battered women. The team noted that there is a pattern of consequences common in the regular, periodic episodes of violence. The female victims often experience great stress and serious emotional trauma and engage in self-destructive activities, including attempts at suicide and excessive alcohol and drug use. Nonetheless, these high-risk women are medicated with depressant drugs. Their medical records describe "vague medical complaints," "suicide," and a variety of "mental illnesses" — as well as treated injuries. It appears that there is a progression of serious emotional debilitation. The study determined that, eventually, one out of three is referred for psychiatric treatment and one in seven finally is committed to a state mental hospital. Others, battered and drugged, succeed in suicide. It is a sad paradox for a woman to seek protection and comfort from the memory of one injury only to find that her refuge becomes a destructive trap.

In many enlightened communities the old, stigmatizing judicial and medical processes are being revised. Help is being offered sensitively in the form of nonthreatening advice and shelters. The slow but sure change in social attitudes has been given impetus by the wholesome candor of respected public figures. And many women have been encouraged to confront the threat, whatever the source, and reach for life.

One hopes that misplaced personal guilt will be reduced as greater understanding lessens public discomfort with these unpleasant realities. But it takes courage to trust others enough to display one's feelings about such experiences. When a person's sense of privacy and wholeness has been so diminished, support from others must be certain and unqualified, for the pain of physical and emotional loss is a tenacious companion. Some survivors will celebrate life. Others will damn its injustice.

In his compelling book *From Here to Eternity*, James Jones penned an excruciating, penetrating monologue for Captain Holmes's wife, Karen. The following excerpts, poignant illustrations of her bitterness toward the events related to her hysterectomy, are reflective of many women's feelings of fear and emptiness as symbolized by that too frequent rite of passage into old age.

"See that?" she said. "You know what that is?... Well, that's a hysterectomy scar," she said. "A hysterectomy is a uterectomy. A uterectomy is an operation in which they excise the uterus. But they call it hysterectomy. You know what hysterectomy comes from, of course? From hysteria. Hysteria and womb and women are synonymous in the medical profession, you know. That's where they get their biggest source of income, you see. You know: stupid women who weep and are very nervous and go to pieces and maybe lose their minds as they approach the change of life ...

"They nod. They soothe you. Mustn't be upset. Be calm. Happens to the best of us. 'Just as I thought,' they say, 'you need a hysterectomy, that's all.' ... But after they sew you up, you suddenly discover that you're not a woman any more. Oh, the outside's still there ... you still look and dress the part of a woman ... even your breasts don't dry up because they've got some little pills to keep the shell acting just the same as though you weren't changed. Hormones, they call them.

"See?" she said, she got a little square green bottle out of the overnight bag she had brought. "You take them every day. The pills you'll never be without. But," she said, "you're still not a woman any more ... you're not anything. You're a gutted shell. What they need to make next is a pill that will give the meaning back, or at least the illusion of the meaning, then you can take two kinds of pills a day and life will be wonderful.

"Maybe," she said, "maybe that's why it is you hunt so hungrily for love, why you have to hunt for it, even though you know they are all secretly laughing at you, winking behind your idealistic romantic back — another neurotic woman at the change of life who wants to change the world and give it love, as if the world ever needed love!

"But love, if you can find it, you think, might give sex meaning — and give you meaning — might even give life meaning. Love is all you've got then — if you can find it."

As most women grow older, they become more frightened. Not only are they in touch with increasing evidence of their own mortality — they ache more, they are needed less, they seem suddenly beset by menopausal symptoms — but they are also confronted with all of the unanswered questions that there was never time enough or courage enough to answer earlier. There are greater possibilities of physical breakdown, of the need for surgery, of becoming widowed. Memories, alone, are painful. The frame of reference is mostly to events and times that have passed, much too quickly. Frequently, the questions women ask are not only "Where did it all go?" but also "Wasn't there something more I intended to do?" and "Is there time?" and "Can I?"

Drug and Alcohol Related Suicides

The greatest percentage of accidental and deliberate suicides that are related to drug and alcohol abuse occurs among mature women. Most of these women were provided with medications to help them "cope." Most of them needed, not prescriptions, but someone to help them find purpose and personal promise. Those who are left alone, confronting isolation from community and family life, especially begin to see themselves as elderly. Those who live on fixed incomes are even more restricted. Sufficient income or not, the constellation of boredom, loneliness, and physical debilitation leads these women to doctors. Accustomed to a lifetime of taking advice and relying on medication, this passive resolution of problems seems appropriate.

Now, in addition to familiar mild sedatives, the doctor may prescribe pain medications, further reducing activity. Like tranquilizers, these narcotic drugs relieve tension but also induce drowsiness and slower respiration. Professional literature calls attention to other side effects of pain killers — namely, chronic constipation, altered kidney function, and a reduction of sex-hormone levels. Unfortunately these symptoms are commonly thought to be associated with aging itself, rather than with the medications given to older people.

The Medicine Routine

Nonetheless, to dull the feelings of worthlessness, alcohol and drugs present comforting appeals to many. Very often, however, this medicated regimen is a contributing, if not the sole, factor of chronic depression and lassitude. In some cases, older women may be encouraged to drink or be given drugs to make them "easier to handle" and less of a problem for those "who care." A well-known film personality recently remarked to me:

> I've been astonished at how often I've been in the company of women and heard them comparing — no, bragging, to each other about the variety of medicines that they must take, and I've wondered why they seem to be in such competition.
>
> One day it finally dawned on me. What they're really saying to each other is: "Look at me. These people care about *me* in all these ways. They're in touch with so many things that hurt *me*, and they're advising, prescribing, and caring."

She was particularly concerned because this pattern, which she had observed in others, was now suddenly an active part of her own widowed mother's life. "There's almost a childish joy in my mother's medicine-taking routine every day, as though each time she takes a pill she is being stroked with loving concern."

In reality, scientific knowledge about aging processes is in its infancy. Myths abound. Frequently diagnoses of depression are the result of medication — including the kinds of medication that are designed to treat the symptoms of depression. Dr. Leo Hollister, a recognized researcher of psycho-active drugs at the VA hospital in Palo Alto, advised in an article in *New England Journal of Medicine* (November 1978) that "patients with depression clearly related to problems of living do not need drug treatment; they tend to tolerate it poorly." This statement was accompanied by other comments on an increasingly popular class of drugs used to treat depression — tricyclic antidepressants. Dr. Hollister referred also to the "confusional reactions . . . most often seen in patients over the age of 40 years," which are worsened "if the patient is also receiving other drugs, such as anti-psychotics . . ." Moreover, he reminds the reader that "mental confusion is common in older patients."

Best estimates suggest that only a fraction over 1 percent of the elderly suffer from the disease, senile dementia. Yet, inappropriate medication, improper doses and combinations, misuse, and unanticipated reactions cause a mistaken perception of the prevalence of "senility" among older people. The worst fears are reinforced by continued acceptance of these attitudes and therapies.

One-fourth of the suicides in the United States are committed by people over sixty-five. In 1977 the Department of Health, Education, and Welfare printed the results of a study on the legal drug use of older Americans, who make up the highest percentage of drug consumers of any age group. As such, the elderly population greatly risks drug dependency, adverse reactions, and drug-induced illnesses.

The report states that 86 percent of people over sixty-five are treated for at least one chronic condition. A variety of drugs are prescribed, many of which are antagonistic, producing a complexity of reactions. Often one drug reduces the metabolism of another, thus extending the latter's intended period of activity overlong. Diet and reduced physical activity frequently cause alterations in the effect as well.

Especially troubling, according to the report, were the differences in health of those who used psychoactive drugs and those who did not. The mood-altering drugs taken were generally sedatives, tranquilizers, and antidepressants, in combination with other prescriptions and over-the-counter preparations. This group of users reported the need for many more prescription drugs overall. By their own descriptions they were certain of their need for these drugs to perform daily activities, but enjoyed life least.

The combined effects of aging, increased incidence of ailments, and a growing number of medications that reduce active functioning may produce a greater sense of impairment and depression. Psychoactive drugs, especially when given in regular adult doses (not adjusted downward for age), frequently produce symptoms identical to pathologies of illness. Unsteadiness, poor coordination, drowsiness, lowered blood pressure, and even increased confusion are not necessarily signals of the coming of life's end. They may be the accompaniments to the use of Thorazine, Stelazine, or Mellaril, commonly prescribed calming drugs for older women. Physicians and patients should become better informed about diagnosing and dosing the aging body. Less is better. It's good to be alive only if you feel alive.

7

Male Doctors, Female Patients

IN RECENT YEARS the list of social or sociable drugs has grown. Apparently the sheer popularity of such drugs makes them acceptable. Increasing numbers of people now consider marijuana one such drug and cocaine another. It appears that among women the drugs most often prescribed by medical caretakers have joined the social list: Tranquilizers, diet pills, and pain remedies are experiences to share, trade, and even desire. Once entrenched, this chemical comforting that characterizes our culture is very difficult to undo.

Along with making social drugs available, our times and technology have also evolved new definitions of socially accepted disease states. These tend to be consonant with cultural expectations. Men are not supposed to complain about pain. They often brag about how strong and resistant they are to suffering and how seldom they see doctors. Women, although biologically stronger, are permitted to experience and describe symptomatic ailments, from headaches, tiredness, aggravation, blues and blahs, to all of those discomforts mysteriously caused by "female plumbing." As we saw earlier, medical marketing ingenuity has elevated these unwanted moods and feelings to disease status and has thrust them into the arena of medical attention — for treatment, but seldom for cure.

"If I Don't Provide It, Someone Else Will"

Doctors have welcomed the pharmaceutical invasion. It has provided them with a virtual chemical cornucopia to modify and mollify the complaints of their largest patient group, women. I once suggested to a woman whose drug-taking troubled me that just as a fever is a signal that infection needs attention, so, too, her moody discomfort might signal a need to examine an underlying problem. She responded, "I don't *need* to be uncomfortable. And besides, the doctor wouldn't give it to me if it weren't for my own good."

Maybe. Here's how one doctor explained it to me:

> I don't know what people expect of us. I spend days, nights, and weeks on end seeing people whose problems range from real disease to nothing but a lot of complaints. I'm not saying that the complaints are unjustified. Those people expect help from me just as much as the ones who would die if I didn't help. But I have to make some distinctions. I can't give them all the same amount of time or concern. The crisis isn't always there, at least not in my judgment.
>
> I've got to be more thorough and careful about the vital signs and records for people who are deathly ill than I do for those who just tell me about where it hurts. I don't even have time to find out all the reasons why. Sometimes life is the reason why. But they wouldn't like to hear that diagnosis, would they? And let's be honest. When a woman comes to me, she doesn't feel well. When she leaves me, she expects to leave with something that will assure that she'll feel better. If I don't provide it for her, you can bet she'll find someone else who will.

Women who have been through the torturous process of overcoming addiction to pills have told me in a variety of ways of their ultimate resentment of the physician who initially offered and then continued to prescribe the very drugs to which they became habituated:

It's such a cop-out. By giving me a pill, he only confirmed that I couldn't really control my own emotions.

Even if I wasn't prepared to tell him what was really troubling me, he could have exhibited some belief in my own strength and just urged me to take hold of my own life better and not let it get me down.

I remember the first night I checked into the halfway house — after I was detoxified. The only thing I really felt was anger. I wanted to write a nasty letter to that doctor. Why did he let me go on for three and a half years with Percodan without once telling me that the warmth and love it made me feel inside was something I ought to try to find outside, that maybe I could, on my own. That night, for the first time in those three and a half years, I wanted him to know how ugly I felt about him and that finally I wasn't dependent on him in any way for a comfortable night's sleep.

A woman whose mother had been addicted to prescription drugs explained her feelings about physicians:

As a general rule, I'm very skeptical of most of them, particularly the mature ones. Even though the current breed — in medical school now — may be a bit different, they still have certain limitations. Through all of those years of training, they don't have to learn how to relate to the human condition. There is no place in medical school for human needs, just physical ailments. They spend sixteen years in school, they've hocked everything, maybe have a wife who's ready to leave, and their greatest need is to clear $70,000 to $80,000. They run their patients in like cattle and pass out the tranquilizers. Their education hasn't taught them differently. They don't think it's a bad thing to do.

And there's more. Suffering women of my mother's generation — and maybe women in general — have very few places to go where they are understood and accepted without a condescending attitude. Whether they say it aloud or not, most doctors are conditioned to think, "Oh, she's just another one of those hysterical women who can't cope."

If they really believe that people develop physical symptoms to get attention, then they ought to give that attention to them. They ought to be able to say, "You're looking for something I can't give you in a bottle, but I'll talk to you and see if we can find a way to resolve your troubles." I might respect doctors again if they developed the wisdom and the courage to do that, not to hook their patients in a professional environment.

A pharmacist friend recalled, with a grimace, her early professional years in a major city hospital. As the chief pharmacist in the outpatient department, she was appalled at the extraordinary numbers of tablets or capsules issued to patients for conditions that were diagnosed as immediate rather than chronic.

I found myself constantly getting on that inside phone and calling those damned doctors. Over and over I had to remind them of the possible danger of many of these drugs if they were taken too often, too much, or too long. They didn't appreciate my second-guessing them one bit. After a while, I simply stopped trying to awaken their consciences and simply made the call to let them know that I was cutting their prescriptions by a third, sometimes in half. I didn't even wait for their pleasure or displeasure to come across the phone. After a while they got to know me and, whether they liked it or not, knowing that had some effect on how much of anything they prescribed.

But what about other hospital pharmacists and other captive patients? Those patients who can afford private doctors are not the only ones susceptible to the overavailability of medical drugs. In some degree, poor people are even more victimized, often by institutional formulas like "more is less": more drugs, fewer visits.

The Double Standard of Health Care

Over the past decade research psychologists have examined the possibility of a double standard of health care, attributable to the affect of sex bias on diagnosis. Their investigations have found that such a double standard does exist; survey after survey reveals that clinical practitioners define healthy men and healthy women quite differently. In addition, the characteristics of "healthy adult" are consonant only with those attributed to males and conflict substantially with traits assigned to healthy females.

Male physicians expect women to be weaker than men — even neurotic. Besides being lead astray by contemporary marketing of panaceas that are graphically designed to address female conditions of distress, doctors have long been imbued with Hippocratic theories and dicta. It is in that venerated tradition — whence comes every physician's promise "never to do harm to anyone" — that the word *hysteria* is defined as "an affliction of the uterus." In the nineteenth century, thousands of clitoral operations were performed on such diseased, "hysterical" women. Antiquated or not, unfortunately the stereotype of the hysterical female remains beneath the cornerstone of contemporary physical and mental health technology and care.

Meanwhile, in their search for meaningful, comfortable, or healthy traditional lives, women have fallen prey to the medical industry's Pandora's box of packaged promises, which all too often contains punishment.

Cruel evidence of this exists in the great numbers of limbless young adults in Europe today, the result of widespread use by pregnant women of the sedative thalidomide. In this country, the inappropriate use of alcohol and medications during pregnancy and even the miracle of painless unconscious delivery are now being seen as having caused deformed or impaired infants. Is it just coincidence that we know of seven million to ten million school children suffering from retardation or brain dysfunction?

How many suicides, ever increasing in number, are accidental toxic reactions to multiple drug use? How many alleged manic-depressives took their lives because they were prescribed and took tranquilizers when a mood-elevator should have been the therapy of choice? How much domestic violence or homicide is related either to the explosion of anger long-repressed by drugs or to drug-induced hostility?

Joanne's Story

Joanne would like to sue someone, or rather, a lot of people in lots of places — but that alone wouldn't solve the problem. So many forces, over so much time, have deprived her of something she cannot regain. What's worse, she has no way to measure its lost value.

Her childhood was stunted by the absence of affection from an alcoholic father and her dread of an erratic mother, whose unknown drug dependency rendered her "a little crazy."

> Can you imagine — for thirty years I never knew. I never had a childhood, never had a mother who was there all along. I spent years working through analysis, trying to overcome that deprivation. All the years I spent running away to survive, she was being dosed — nearly to death — and I didn't know. It's bizarre. The whole thing feels like a conspiracy.

About five years ago, Joanne decided to make a quick trip to the northwestern state where her mother lived alone in the house where Joanne had spent her childhood. "Something about the lateness of my mother's calls and the way she sounded made me worry." When she arrived, she saw all of the symptoms of deterioration and disorientation. "Packages of unopened groceries on the porch and in the house, unread newspapers piled up along the front steps — everything was a mess. It also became evident that she had her days and nights reversed."

Joanne quickly called her mother's doctor and, after describing her mother's state of confusion, incoherent mumbling, and lack of coordination, an ambulance was sent to take her to the hospital. While her mother was being admitted, Joanne was shocked to hear the head nurse refer to her mother as a drug addict. After the admission procedures were completed and her mother was taken to a medical care unit in the psychiatric wing, Joanne confronted the doctor: "You know, my mother needs psychiatric help, she's always had a mental and emotional problem." Since she had never met this doctor, she felt the need to explain her mother's past years of instability. (Their family doctor, the man who delivered Joanne and was her mother's friend and personal physician, had recently retired.) The doctor responded with quiet firmness.

> No, she doesn't just need psychiatric care. There's nothing wrong with her mind except too many pills. She's suffering from a toxic overdose and I've ordered medical withdrawal. She's now having her system pumped. Then I'll put her on decreasing doses of Thorazine.

During the night, her mother became totally irrational. She began hallucinating and having convulsions. Apparently, even this doctor had no idea of the level of drug use she had reached. Incredulous, Joanne was convinced her mother really was an addict. But, for how long? And had anyone else known about it? She checked with the hospital administrator and discovered that, during the previous couple of years, her mother had been a regular visitor to the emergency room.

Her friends had brought her there when she suffered from overdoses. She would have her stomach pumped and then leave, never staying at the hospital longer than two days. The records indicated that she would return home and the cycle would begin again.

Joanne spent the next few days wandering around the house, trying to put it in order and searching her memory for clues to this newly discovered truth. Wherever she looked or reached she found pill bottles, an unbelievable assortment of five hundred containers, with dates going back as far as twenty years. And there were tissues everywhere, all crumpled up. As she cleaned the house, she accumulated bags and mounds of clean, wadded tissues. Sudenly she recalled,

Of course, every picture I conjure up, as far back as my memory serves, my mother always had a handkerchief or a tissue in her hand. It was always there. My God, now it made sense. They always had pills in them!

I always knew, as did everyone else, that she was constantly taking medication. She made a big deal about it. She would take out a bottle and announce, at any time, in any setting, "time for my tranquilizer," or "time for my medicine." And it seemed to make sense. We all knew that she had had a lot of surgery when I was very young, gall bladder and other operations. Everyone understood and agreed that she did the best she could, considering the pain and her emotional conditions. I believed it. And in her way, those ritual announcements were designed to make us all approve of her medical controls, even to admire her open concern about her otherwise unstable condition.

Joanne went on to recall odd behavior that had punctuated her teen years.

Mother used to have regular seizures, they were called partial seizures. All at once I now realized that they had had a clear schedule. Each was precipitated by the threat of a change. Any time my brother or I planned a vacation, a visit to friends, a move to college, any movement away from her, she would get sick, faint, and when revived, have amnesia. It was a cry for help and all she got was more medicine. In the morning, afternoon, and evening, she took the prescribed amount from bottles, and when no one was looking, her helpful handkerchiefs disguised the pills she needed to fill other voids, all day and all night.

Joanne started charting her mother's habit, using the dates on the prescription containers as a calendar, a chronicle of her mother's life, which also documented the history of pharmaceutical marketing. Every change in mood-altering therapy filled the table. Sedatives — from barbiturates to minor tranquilizers — amphetamines and their derivatives, antidepressants, mood-elevators, and estrogen compounds. Joanne began grouping them by dates to see if they coincided with difficult events that she could remember. The greatest profusion seemed to correlate with her father's death and with the tragic accident that took her brother's life three years later. During those periods the prescriptions seemed to come in pairs, at least. (She even found a dozen or more bottles of drugs issued in the names of her mother's friends.) The newest prescriptions had been ordered by her mother's new doctor.

I went to the pharmacies that had dispensed these drugs for so many years. I needed to find out how she could have gotten so many for so long. They accepted no responsibility. They said, "We don't regulate, we just act on the doctor's orders. She had standing prescriptions. Either she called us or the nurse would. All we do is fill prescriptions and sell medicine. We don't make judgments or offer advice."

Joanne tracked down the retired doctor. She challenged him: "How can you justify these prescriptions? There are even double prescriptions. Here — Equanil — two bottles, each with one hundred fifty-milligram tablets. Here are two bottles authorized by your office on the same day. One, a prescription, and one that you gave her directly. How can you explain that?"

He apologized but said that there was very little else he could have done. He insisted,

> I tried everything. Early in the sixties I worked so hard to get her off the barbiturates, but it wasn't easy. I finally got her to use Librium instead, as a transition. I told her that I didn't want to give her anymore. But she pleaded with me. We were friends, and each time she gave me another reason, another excuse. No one knew better than I how much pain she felt. You see, I myself spent many years fighting with addiction, taking cures, and suffering. I understood your mother and I cared about her pain. I couldn't leave her on a psychiatric ward. When she screamed, "Get me out of here," I was helpless. I didn't know how else to help.

During the next several days as Joanne checked on her mother's condition, she continued to dwell in the agonizing past, on a lifetime of misinterpretation. She remembered all the years of tiptoeing around her mother's moods and planning her own escape, each day more certain that her survival depended on leaving. Only now did she realize that she had been skirting only a facade — this schizophrenic, often paranoid personality — an unrecognizable being, driven by and to drugs. There had never been a normal discussion, conversation, sharing of experiences or friendship. Every such effort was inevitably shattered by an inexplicable mood shift. The longer she thought about it, the more certain she perceived the enormity of the collusion.

> My brother and I lived with two cripples, and only they knew the whole secret. My father was too smart not to

know, and he never said a word, except to remind us to "take care of mother, be good to her." Just as my mother would say, "Your father is sick, you need to take care of him."

Joanne was simultaneously contrite and frustrated, remembering the years she had spent in psychotherapy, talking about how she had been cheated of her childhood needs, never getting love, always having to give it, without a reservoir to draw on. Now with dismay she recalls that her fantasies of escape were enhanced by her father's urging her to move on, to excel, to have a career. Those brief, sober talks were as close as he ever came to expressing fatherly love and concern, and so they were immensely important to her. She could rationalize any uncertainty about leaving home by acting on what her father "expected" of her. She wanted his approval, if she couldn't have affection. Whose best interests were really being served? Her distance from them simply provided more time to leave the conspiracy of silence intact and gave their lives more space in which to flounder.

After about five days, when her mother's withdrawal dosage had been greatly reduced, she started agitating to leave the hospital. The doctor called Joanne and asked her to come immediately. When she arrived, she found her mother adamant, dressed in her coat and waiting at the door, saying, "I'm going with you. You're taking me out of here." Joanne looked in panic to the doctor and hoped for assistance. Her mother, staring hard, continued: "You're trying to kill me. You'd like to have all my money. I want you to take me out of here. Now! If you don't, I'll hate you for the rest of my life."

In a barely audible whisper, Joanne pleaded, "No. Please, mother, no. I can't take you from here, not yet."

Mercifully, the doctor interceded. He looked straight at her mother and said, "You are a drug addict and you need help.

You are going to stay here. I'm advising your daughter to get a court order to keep you here."

Joanne reached out to hold on to him as one would grab a life line.

> Oh, thank you. Help me to do what needs to be done. Doctors have not listened to me in years. They haven't even talked to me about what was wrong with my mother. I'm not sure what I should do — what's right to do. What will happen if I let her have her way, if I let her leave?

He responded quickly, "She'll die — and very soon. Her system cannot take any more drugs."

Joanne looked from the doctor to her mother. She saw the terror of what it means to be an addict, to be separated from drugs. Her mother's face was contorted by anger and fear. Joanne was relieved to go home.

For the next two weeks, Joanne was told not to visit the hospital. The medical team worked with her mother, around the clock, trying to stabilize her convulsions. When she was not physically ill, her mother devised one ruse after another in order to be released. None of them worked. To assure that no fabrications would be helped by friends, Joanne alerted all of her mother's likely collaborators that this deadly game was ended. She dealt with many outraged women, some of whom had been members of the drug-trading network. She took abuse, accepted charges that she didn't care about her mother and was mistreating her. Certain that she had made a correct life-and-death decision, she remained firm and warned them to stay away. She advised them that, like it or not, they would have to accept her determination that her mother would remain in the hospital. She warned that any contrary actions would be dealt with in a court of law.

The more she talked about legal action, the more it seemed a useful thing to do. She wondered if such a suit wouldn't focus attention on all the cracks in the medical care system, on the responsibility of doctors, and the role of pharmacists, on emergency room practices, on hospitals and record keeping, even on the questionable safety factor of approved drugs. Her interest provoked inquiry. But it collided with existing state law. She found that only the aggrieved party, in this case her mother, could bring such a suit. Next-of-kin were disallowed.

Several weeks later, when Joanne was permitted to visit with her mother, she told her of the bitter legal pill she had been forced to swallow and why. Her mother was incensed at the notion that Joanne would have considered taking such action. In addition, for all that she had been through and even all that it meant for her future, she had been an addict long enough to know that at some point there are so many to blame, that no single person can be blamed. What's more, she still believed that everyone who kept her "secret" did so only out of concern and kindness — either they didn't know any better, or it was better that they didn't know. Joanne's mother volunteered to join a chemical dependency unit program attached to the hospital. For the first time in almost thirty years, she admitted that she had a drug problem and was willing to remedy it.

Everyone on the medical staff cautioned Joanne not to put too much faith in her mother's resolve. "After so many years, there may be only a 20 percent chance of recovery." Joanne stayed close for several more weeks. She and her mother would walk the halls together and talk about things that they had never shared before. Joanne was startled the day her mother talked about her brother. She asked, "By the way, where is your brother these days?" And she listened to Joanne. In that hallway, there was finally the full recognition that, seven years earlier, her son had been killed.

By the time Joanne's mother left the dependency unit, she had experienced the pain of separation from a lifetime of drugs, as well as the grief (delayed for seven years) of the loss of her son. At various stages in her therapy, Joanne's mother would discuss some of the anguish she had experienced early in her life: how she had been terrorized by her husband's alcoholism; how, with two small children, no job skills, and no family of her own, she had felt trapped, with no place and no one to turn to. She asked her daughter how much she blamed her for not leaving him. Joanne could not tell her of the shame she felt for having loved her father in spite of his problem while believing that her mother was a weak, unredeemable failure.

The most compelling conversation for Joanne was the one in which her mother expressed the horror and utter hopelessness she had experienced in her addiction. She described the fear of discovery; the weeks and months of making repeated decisions to stop; how she would cut pills in half and pray to God to stop her. But there had been no one to help her, no place to hide, and no place to cry.

After several months of treatment, Joanne's mother was released from the hospital joyfully exclaiming, "For the first time in my life, I'm free — for the first time in my life." She said to Joanne, "I know I must have said some awful things to you, and I don't expect you to understand. After all this time, I don't even expect you to forgive me. I just hope you'll forget them."

Joanne has not really been able to forget what she has struggled so hard to remember, to sort out, and to accept. She recognizes the enormity of what her mother has indeed overcome. Five years have passed without pills. Mother and daughter maintain a more pleasant relationship, but it's difficult because it has so little history, practically no nostalgia.

Joanne's mother was surely victimized, but now she is free. Joanne, on the other hand, still has her injured feelings, her empty places, anger, confusion, and also her guilt — for not being able to love this woman, this stranger, this mother she never had.

8

The Drugs and How They Work

"SOCIAL" DRUGS, such as alcohol, cigarettes, and coffee, are all psychoactive, and many people become dependent upon them to one degree or another. Without our being aware of it, simple daily habits can contribute to nervous-system confusion. Many of the foods and liquids that we ingest and the remedies that we buy without prescription contain agents that interact with prescribed drugs and may enhance or diminish their effectiveness. For example, the caffeine in coffee is a stimulant, whereas various cold remedies containing antihistamines are depressants. Some prescribed and over-the-counter drugs combine both stimulants and depressants.

Ephedrine, a stimulant in decongestant remedies, may cause a rapid rise in blood pressure and, consequently, severe headaches when taken with certain antidepressants. Likewise, because of their particular chemical composition, strong cheeses and herring cause a similar reaction when eaten in conjunction with such antidepressants as Nardil and Marplan. Alcohol combined with antidepressants causes deep sedation and a severe drop in body temperature. Any sleeping pill, tranquilizer, or antihistamine used along with such antidepressants as Elevil will exaggerate the sedative effects on body function, producing respiratory depression, dizziness, drowsiness, or fainting. Drugs prescribed to thin blood and reduce clotting should not be taken with aspirin or any other analgesic. Likewise, the combination of thyroid preparations or cholesterol-lowering medication with any analgesic may incite internal bleeding and possible hemorrhaging. Also, anticoagulants are counteracted by the ingestion of large portions of green, leafy vegetables.

In addition, various external circumstances can act on our bodies and cause internal responses. Weather, anxiety, excitement, all interact with drug chemistry and might produce unexpected effects.

In spite of the absence of complete and absolute information about distribution and all actions of mood-altering drugs, they have become a mainstay of medical practice. Certain general characteristics are known about the effects of these drugs. While each category may be distinctive, all alter the user's state of awareness. These drugs are intended either to elevate or decrease functional activity and, simultaneously, may affect pain, mood, or tension. All of the promotional emphasis notwithstanding, there is clear empirical evidence that dependence may develop with all central nervous system drugs (particularly depressants), when taken for extended periods of time.

Depressants

Drugs that are designed to act as depressants of the central nervous system inhibit or block the transmission of neurological signals and so suppress many physical and cell functions throughout the body. Less reported and even less understood is the effect described as "paradoxical excitement." In these situations, the opposite of the intended sedative result occurs.

Among prescribed drugs, minor tranquilizers are already

the drugs most frequently used in combination with other drugs as well as alcohol. The effects of some of them, like Miltown and Equanil, are hard to distinguish from the stronger sedatives. These minor tranquilizers, like the barbiturates, compete with alcohol for the same liver enzymes in order to be metabolized and eliminated from the body. Thus, when these drugs are combined with alcohol they remain in the blood stream in dangerously high amounts and for a longer time. Consequently, the use of multiple depressants is very common in accidental or deliberate suicides.

Barring that fatal result, certain of these drugs have other dangerous characteristics. They are stored in the body's fatty tissues and do not leave the system easily. Consequently, even if a person stops taking medication that causes an unpleasant effect, that discomfort may not be fully relieved immediately. Since the drug is stored in the body tissue, it will continue to be released into the system for some time, continuing complications. Depending on levels of accumulation, residues may affect coordination and reaction time for as many as eight days after use. Driving a car during drug use may be no more hazardous than it is days later. Since women generally have more fatty (adipose) tissue throughout their bodies than men, the amount of drug retention and redistribution may be greater for them. And keep in mind that the brain is the single largest fatty organ in the body.

The most popular minor tranquilizers in recent years — Librium and Valium — are pharmacologically not very different from their predecessors. In addition to acting as sedatives, however, these drugs also relax muscles and have somewhat better anticonvulsant qualities. Many of these drugs are also used extensively in the treatment of alcoholism because they reduce the unpleasant effects of abstinence. In too many cases, the "cure" has become the problem.

Many alcoholism specialists refer to sedative and tranquilizer medications as solid alcohol.

Stimulants

On the other end of the drug spectrum, the use of stimulants makes it difficult to properly stabilize life and behavior. More times than not, users develop erratic patterns of daily medication, alternating between stimulation and sedation. Many people find themselves behaving in a manner akin to schizophrenia upon cessation of these drugs and are often hospitalized with that diagnosis. Some cases are so severe that convulsions and a sense of persecution occur along with illusions that verge on hallucination.

Although it is possible that some stimulants decrease the lethal depressant qualities of alcohol, this is not generally true. Nor is it always a desirable antidote. Some cases suggest that the combination produces excessive excitability and may even induce convulsions. And there is some evidence that changes in brain chemistry may remain when the drug use has ceased.

Whatever else they do, all these classes of drugs alter the central nervous system, which is a combination of the spinal cord and the brain. Any drug capable of influencing the mind consequently affects one's physical state. In turn, alterations in physical function trigger a mental response.

There is no mechanism more complex than the human brain. The working relationship of approximately ten billion neurons and even more cells is involved in the human maze known as the central nervous system. Think of the brain as the control center of a major communications network — the nervous system. All voluntary and involuntary impulses are transmitted from the control center through the communication lines (nerves). They go to and from the brain, meet at various critical points, and branch out to perform and inspire all the obvious and subtle functions throughout the body: They control more than five hundred muscles, which affect all possible movement (of limbs, eyes, eyelids, mouth, and even the ability to shape words with the tongue); respiration and digestion; hormonal balance and ovarian functions; skin texture; and even what we remember. All of these are determined by connected networks that begin with the brain and are part of the head-to-toe complex of the nervous system — which we so blithely depress or excite with drugs.

During times of stress, when there is an implosion of events or stimuli, it is perfectly natural for healthy human beings to respond in instinctive, often primitive ways. Rather than stimulating self-blame or guilt over seemingly irrational behavior, quick, even emotional reactions might be viewed as appropriate responses to basic brain orders. Once again, history is instructive. The oldest brain formations produced "fight or flight" reactions, often referred to as survival instincts. Only later did the human brain develop emotional control centers for evaluation of those responses (allowing reason to be superimposed). But that primary system is still the quickest to react to danger or even perceived danger. Often the response is so quick that the higher sense of rationality has no time to intervene.

A complex life and time may make it impossible to separate, resolve, or comprehend sufficiently the sheer number and close sequence of threatening pressures. Instead our mind and body may react to the preponderant weight, even without thought. How often have each of us, with dismay, worried (after the fact) about "losing my temper," or "not knowing what got into me"? Have no fear — such spontaneous behavior is not necessarily "neurotic." It may signify a healthy response of the oldest brain process known, not a tranquilizer deficiency. The time to worry is when the mind or body, or both of them, have been so affected by chemicals

DRUG CHART: *What to Expect*

	Dependence Potential	Effective Time	Rx Uses	Effects Likely	Overdose Symptoms	Withdrawal Conditions
NARCOTIC and SYNTHETIC ANALGESICS (pain relievers) Morphine Dilaudid Percodan Nisentil Codeine Demerol Darvon Lomotil Leritene Dolene SK-65 Prinadol Talwin	high (except for Codeine, which is moderate)	3–6 hours	analgesia, antitussive, antidiarrheal	euphoria, drowsiness, nausea, respiratory depression	slow & shallow breathing, clammy, coma	irritability, chills, sweats, tremors, cramps, no appetite
BARBITURATES, SEDATIVES, and TRANQUILIZERS Thorazine Stelazine Mellaril Nembutal Amytal Butisol Seconal Mebaral Luminal Gemonil Ipral Nodular Tuinal Doriden Quaalude Tranxene Miltown Equanil Meprospan Valium Librium Placidyl Beta-Chlor Vistaril Dalmane Triclos Serax Milpath Solacen Tybatran Atarex	moderate to high, with high tolerance (need for increased levels)	1–16 hours	sedation, sleep, convulsion muscle relaxation anti-anxiety	slurred speech, disorientation poor coordination (similar to drunkenness)	weak and rapid pulse, cold and clammy skin, shallow breathing, coma, possible death	anxiety, delirium, convulsions, insomnia, tremors, abnormal brain waves
(The most widely used, legal depressant drug is alcohol. In addition to whiskey, beer, wines, and cordials, alcohol is used in over-the-counter medications and as a solvent in some prescriptions.)	Active sedative elements remain in the blood for varying lengths of time. Those in the Gemonil and Luminal groups have "half-lives" of up to 96 hours; Amytal, Butisol, and Nembutal remain for no more than 42 hours. Dalmane, Valium, and Librium classes leave residues up to 8 days.					
AMPHETAMINES and AMPHETAMINE-LIKE COMPOUNDS Eskatrol Obetrol Benzedrine P-A-D Tabs Ionamin Norodin Sanorex Voranil Dexedrine Biphetamine Preludin Tenuate Bamadex Phentermine Methadrine Pre-Sate	generally high (less for very mild diet pills)	2–4 hours	hyperkinesis, narcolepsy, appetite control	increased pulse and blood pressure, insomnia, excitation, dilated pupils, no appetite	agitation, rise in body temperature, hallucinations, convulsions, possible death	depression, apathy, disorientation, extended periods of sleep

DEPRESSANTS (first two groups) — STIMULANTS (amphetamines group) that they don't distinguish or act on signals, and protective instincts may be muted; or when simple events are always computed as overwhelming.

Those too-available, fixed-dose, mood-altering drugs are universally prescribed for men and women — without acknowledgment of differences in anatomy, environment, nutrition, long-term prognoses, and female cyclical hormonal changes as indicators for dosage variation. Instead of relying solely on the industry-prepared *Physician's Desk Reference,* it would be useful for doctors to reflect on the efficacy of any chemical interference. One rule of thumb should be kept in mind: When a drug is taken for relief or adjustment of one symptom, whether pain or mood, its action will likely have many, more comprehensive effects on the body.

At a recent meeting with four physician-pharmacologists at the Food and Drug Administration, I asked, "What happens when a woman swallows either a chemical depressant or stimulant? Do you know where all of it goes and by what route? And whatever the drug's intended purpose, do you know how much and when one affected system triggers activity in another functional area?"

Their responses made it clear that, for all the headway that scientists and highly specialized physicians have made, there are still many more frontiers of knowledge that have not yet been crossed. They admitted that there are no certain answers to those basic, critical questions: "If we, any of us, could find the answers, we would earn a Nobel Prize." Yet drug marketing and labeling decisions are made even with limited insight — and these public health officials are concerned about it. They are troubled by the proliferation of mood-altering drugs and the increasing likelihood of unforeseen, multidrug-induced illness: "No one knows for sure the long-range, cumulative effect or damage to the generally healthy human condition."

9

The Big Mood-Altering Business

LIKE MANY OTHER service industries whose fortunes rest on a supply-and-demand ratio, the search for better health has created an enormous marketplace. Strong professional and economic relationships have been forged among various sectors of the health field. They share many interests and prospects. From time to time, government and public-interest investigations have raised doubts about the propriety of certain political and investment partnerships between pharmacists, physicians, researchers, and manufacturers, as well as their connections with regulatory bodies. The undisclosed, unchecked power that these elements of the health industry wield collectively is awesome. Together they determine the emphasis, costs, quality, and availability of all aspects of health care. This alliance, along with the influence each segment exerts on the other, is a major consideration in some of the underlying causes for the drug destiny of women.

Whether or not official action will ever effectively disconnect these myriad interlocking mechanisms depends to some degree on an active, public, survival consciousness. We need first of all to cast light onto these collegial corners of commerce for a better understanding of these unseen forces. In doing so we should be able to mitigate the guilt we have felt for actions that are not entirely within our own control.

I am certain that some of the hazards consumers face are a direct result of a lack of checks and balances within a system we depend on to provide us with safe and effective therapy. Mistakenly, we act on the notion that nothing arrives on the American food or drug market unless it is entirely safe and is so approved by the various guardians of the public health. But who renders those judgments and on what basis?

Industry-Government Incest

The topmost levels of the Food and Drug Administration have often been peopled by those who were just previously employed by some of the major pharmaceutical manufacturing companies. Conversely, many of the decision makers who began their service within the regulatory agency later established new careers as highly paid officers or board members of pharmaceutical companies. There has been in fact a constant exchange between the leading representatives of the profession and the various monitoring and lobbying bodies that affect its interests. Such interdependency exists between many sectors within the health care system. Some of these relationships may be antithetical to good health.

Consider, what is the effect on consumers when:

• prescribing physicians own retail pharmacies or clinics?

• a doctor's philanthropic reputation is enhanced by the gifts a manufacturer makes, in his name, to medical schools in return for filling out reports on company salesmen?

• medical societies invest pension and other funds in pharmaceutical stock?

• an "objective" scientific researcher, assigned to assess the safety and usefulness of a drug, is also the recipient of the manufacturer's funds for other academic research?

• after accepting and dispensing "free clinical trial goods" from a friendly sales representative, the physician sees an adverse drug reaction, which he may choose to report or ignore?

How may these results affect our protective Food and Drug Administration? The FDA is a passive government agency that acts on information it receives, voluntarily in most instances, from the medical field, the manufacturers, the physicians, hospitals, and so on. The FDA has a limited mandate to monitor. While they urge that reports of toxicity or any adverse reactions be made, they have no authority to require it. It is voluntary. A preponderance of evidence is generally necessary to cause the FDA to take remedial actions, whether in regard to labeling or standards of use.

The FDA's system of regulation has come under attack over and over by the industry as well as consumer groups. From time to time, the love feast dissolves into a serious contest of "It's not my fault." For example, in 1973 Henry Simmons, then the director of the FDA's Bureau of Drugs, delivered a lengthy statement before Senator Gaylord Nelson's Subcommittee on Monopoly in response to criticisms being leveled at his agency. He countercharged that any betrayal of the public trust should be laid at the feet of the drug companies, not the FDA.

Simmons pointed out that after the 1962 laws were passed (the Kefauver-Harris amendments) the FDA, in conjunction with the National Academy of Sciences, did a review of the effectiveness of 4300 drugs that had been approved for distribution in the previous twenty-four years. That review found that only *two out of every five* drugs were clearly effective. In addition, they found that the manufacturers had made 16,000 various claims of therapeutic value for those drugs. The evidence was that only *one in five* of those claims was defensible.

His testimony went on to note that the overprescription of drugs by physicians has created a major health hazard. Simmons argued with the industry's complaints that too much regulation was stifling new drugs for Americans. The number of truly new drugs introduced in the United States had long remained stable — for the previous twenty-two years, only between five and seven new compounds a year. He explained that the rest of the drugs that were introduced were nothing more than recombinations or minor changes in already existing drugs. Industry's criticism of government control has often enjoyed wide citizen support, particularly the claim that the American system of drug control has distorted the cost of research, necessitating the shift of new inquiry to foreign countries. The implication that millions of Americans suffering from many common diseases are being denied these new developments is compelling, but arguable.

According to Simmons, "The pharmaceutical industry remains one of the healthiest and most profitable industries of the nation." Moreover, he submitted information that in 1969 and 1970, of the hundreds of drugs offered by pharmaceutical companies to the regulatory agencies of France, England, and Germany, only four of them were marketed in those three nations, whose regulations are clearly not as rigid — according to the industry.

There is such an aura of secrecy at the FDA regarding necessary scientific tests (which the agency calls, and the industry agrees is, "proprietary data") that one is led to suspect that private interest is more important than scientific considerations at the agency. A 1971 report to the commissioner of food and drugs by an ad hoc advisory committee known as the Ritts committee concluded that "scientific evidence was awarded a low status among the factors in FDA decision making and that in the absence of adequate science, politics governed the decision results."

The Secret History of "the Pill"

In an article in 1975, Anita Johnson, then with Ralph Nader's Health Research Group, criticized the FDA's secrecy. While noting that most toxic drug information was kept from the public by the FDA, she further stated that no one except the drug companies, who submit that information, have access to it, and the practical result is that only those companies are in a position to negotiate with the FDA for lenient decisions and favorable operating policies. More importantly, inaction or delay (common in the process between the industry and the FDA) results in often dangerous drugs remaining on the market even after there is a body of evidence of either their ineffectiveness or their lack of safety.

For example, birth control pills were first tested and approved in the late 1950s for general use in 1960. Although rumors about blood clotting problems among Pill users began shortly thereafter, it took five years of increasing controversy to stimulate a Senate review. Those hearings examined the original Puerto Rican study on which FDA approval was based. For the first time it was found that only 132 women were used in the test group and for only one year. Among that group at least two or three unexplained deaths occurred.

From the 1950s until June of 1970 the number of women using the Pill had grown from the original 132 to 8.5 million. The FDA finally agreed that a warning should be attached to the birth control package for consumers as well as for physicians. Very recently, different dosages and formulations of these medications have been made available and are said to reduce the risk to users. However, the possible jeopardy of these new combinations may not be seen for some time. Even when new dangers are reported, official warnings are slow in coming. Remedies are unevenly applied and remain subject to political and private-interest pressures.

It is interesting to note that in Britain with a national

health system, and quicker, more uniform means of education to physicians, there has been an enormous voluntary reduction in the numbers of women still using this form of contraception.

One of the measures that the FDA relies upon is a ratio of "benefit to risk" But what does this judgment constitute? Does it rely on a percentage of population use? What is an acceptable level of new disease or death? And who determines a drug's benefits and risks? The interested manufacturer? A passive government agency? Or the consumers who may finally be statistics? The plea-bargaining system prevails behind closed doors.

Successful negotiation, which results in broad language of acceptable use for a new drug, is a *critical* first step in the profit-making possibilities of any manufacturer. It is the beginning of the artful campaign that affects acceptance by physicians and the public and so determines major use or not.

The Testing Process: Whose Benefit, What Risks?

At the outset the manufacturer sponsors an application to the FDA to begin animal testing for a new chemical that it maintains will eventually be useful to humans. Initially, all that has to be asserted is that this new agent has promise of bearing some medicinal properties. Clearly, early in the application process the company has to prepare a description of some disease state or designate a condition or function that will justify the lengthy process. In the laboratory, animals are used to determine whether the effects of the drug are desirable, what effects it has, and what the assumed safe (versus poisonous) dosages may be for humans.

This entire preclinical testing phase is not regulated on site by the FDA. It is considered simply a preliminary process to demonstrate a reason to begin testing drugs on humans. That next phase follows the manufacturer's completion of a required form that includes such information as the composition of the drug, what it is derived from, how it is made. The manufacturer also submits the results of the animal studies to assure that enough testing has been performed and describes the plan for human testing. Once approved, "clinical" testing is begun, ostensibly to better determine the dosage level. Here again, the manufacturer hires his own clinical investigator. Thus far, there is no "guardian" presence.

Clinical testing involves the use of this new chemical on patients who have the "disease" that this new drug will treat. At this stage, both effectiveness and side effects have to be observed. Finally, private physicians are given the new drug for their patients' use. Their reports go back to the manufacturer and are supposed to record adverse side effects. Only after the final phase of human research is completed and the safety and effectiveness of dosage levels are asserted does the sponsor submit an application to market the new drug. Proposed labels accompany this application along with a description of the manufacturing process, samples of the drug, and a suggested process of distribution. Finally, at this stage, the FDA's Bureau of Drugs makes a determination regarding the benefits of the drug and its relationship to possible risks. A difficult judgment, no doubt, since no drug is completely free from risk.

After a drug has been marketed, if a dispute arises regarding any of the factors claimed earlier by the manufacturer, a lengthy process of hearings and even court cases may ensue. In each case the FDA has been the recipient of industry determinations and has only that limited information and observational contrary data on which to base its arguments.

The industry is in a very strong position from the first to determine all information relating to the drug, including states of mind that are deemed dysfunctional and hence a disease. Any desirable alteration in the existing condition, which they have designated as unhealthy, winds up on the label as appropriate use for the new drug. Such information also becomes part of the *Physician's Desk Reference*, the bible of practitioners, which is designed and paid for by the manufacturers whose products are described therein.

Enormous budgets are developed for the promotion and sales of these new drugs to doctors and other health professionals. Salesmen are given careful instructions on the company's short- and long-term promotional policies for each drug. Thus, depending on the pattern of use and public acceptability of a drug, the representative's emphasis might change, as an ex-salesman explained in Chapter 1. Carefully designed information is put in the messages that medical schools, pharmacists, and physicians receive through brochures, journals, and conversations with the army of salesmen whose successes are measured by orders.

I have been told by various less circumspect pharmaceutical sales people about the information they shared with each other in order to better understand their respective companies' strategems and purposes. They would pass on names of those physicians referred to as "reporting doctors." Reporting doctors are telephoned regularly by private survey companies under contract to pharmaceutical manufacturers and are asked which salesmen visited and which drugs were discussed.

One sales representative told me the following:

> There were reporting physicians who would fill out a form that included in what order the products were discussed. We were graded as having given an excellent, good, or poor presentation, and the doctor wrote down what samples were left. I gradually learned who the reporting physicians were. Often my friendly doctors would let me fill out the form, grade myself, and I would make sure I put down the products I was supposed to be promoting, and in the cor-

rect order. The reasons the doctor would do this is that the company would send his medical school ten dollars for each report.

The Drug Companies and the Medical Schools

The cost of a medical education continues to skyrocket. Gift supplies, from medical kits and stethoscopes to specialized textbooks, are among the various ways the industry ingratiates itself with students. Other friendly assistance may take the form of summer-job offers or grants for research projects. Beginning with the first year of medical school, unsolicited fliers, newsletters, and journals are received daily. Personal visits and congenial relationships are established by industry salesmen who may provide supplies for campus parties. It is fair to say that most medical students, interns, and residents spend more time with the representatives and products of specific manufacturers than they do in required courses in pharmacology. Although most medical schools now require some basic instruction in limited aspects of this science, it is insufficient. There is no real effort made to assure that physicians will become knowledgeable prescribers independent of industry's private interests.

The working relationship between the medical schools, colleges of pharmacy, and the manufacturers of medical devices and therapeutic drugs has grown increasingly significant. The industry also assists the increasingly economically pressed universities and colleges with regular grants, scholarship funds, equipment, and lecturers and even provides, on a collaborative basis, continuing education courses for which practicing physicians and pharmacists receive credit.

One such recent course, prepared with the assistance of the National Institute on Drug Abuse, depends on a textbook that describes particular properties of commonly prescribed, dangerous drugs. In addition, the book contains not only the quiz to be completed for earned credit, but also an answer sheet supplying the proper responses to that test. By simply filling out the required forms and submitting them to the medical school associated with this effort, a practicing physician may be awarded four continuing-education credits as well as a certificate — the Physician's Recognition Award — attesting to this education attainment, by the American Medical Association. Other "courses" are available on accredited cruise ships and at family resorts. There are many ways to overcome a physician's possible disinclination to continue academic study, and clearly there are many reasons for patients to remain somewhat less than awed by a proliferation of continuing education awards that may appear on office walls.

The Valium Public-Relations Caper

Perhaps the most recent blatant example of questionable relationships between industry, academia, professionals, and government is epitomized by a glossy news kit prepared in a tasteful, sturdy gray and white. On the cover the title reads "The Consequences of Stress: The Medical and Social Implications of Prescribing Tranquilizers." Affixed to one corner is the seal of Cornell University. The kit contains a letter from a major public relations company in New York announcing the convening of an editorial board of seven eminent teaching physicians who "will disseminate information on stress and its management over the next three years." The executive editor of the materials to be developed under this title is Dr. Theodore Cooper, currently dean of the Cornell Medical College. Just prior to becoming dean, Dr. Cooper was the assistant secretary for health in the Department of Health, Education, and Welfare.

A further look raises questions. Although promising a ten-point subject area that will take three years for review, analysis, and subsequent public and professional education, the press releases conflict with the projected openness of examination. One press release has Dr. Cooper explaining that choice of treatment depends on the doctor's evaluation. Moreover, "drug therapy may be the fastest and most effective way to relieve pain symptoms for the patient who is overwhelmed by the consequence of stress." Cooper adds, "The editorial board will examine the anti-anxiety drugs, such as Valium (the trade name for a Hoffman-LaRoche product) and the other benzodiazepine tranquilizers that are 'appropriate and effective.' The problem," says Dr. Cooper, "is not tranquilizer abuse; *it is patient misuse of alcohol and other drugs that act on the central nervous system with tranquilizers*" (my italics).

The second press release, entitled "The Proper Use of Tranquilizers: A Personal Responsibility," hones in on current media criticisms that have been leveled against tranquilizer drugs. According to Dr. Cooper, "it is not tranquilizers as such that have caused the problems but rather it is their misuse; there are relatively few problems with tranquilizers, such as Valium and other benzodiazepines, when one considers the number of people taking them."

Excerpts from the balance of this press release are a fascinating glimpse into a prospective inquiry about which its chairman seems to have drawn conclusions without the benefit of his colleagues. Dr. Cooper states:

> Studies show that the preponderance of all emergency room visits involving psychotrophic or anti-anxiety drugs also involve alcohol. Likewise, when you hear of a person who has gotten into trouble with tranquilizers, you will most often find that alcohol is the villain.

> Valium is the benzodiazepine tranquilizer people are most familiar with. Because it is the most widely prescribed tranquilizer, it has become controversial. In reality, however, the scientific and clinical literature has established its safety

and reliability... Following the doctor's instruction and assuming the proper responsibility for proper use of tranquilizers the patient can be better assured that they provide maximum benefits with a minimum amount of risks.

What began as a scholarly investigation into the underlying causes of stress (which is declared by the program sponsors to be the reason for more than 50 percent of patient visits to physicians) has become an intensive discussion of tranquilizer therapy, singling out Valium in particular. The questions of safety and effectiveness have already been resolved by a man whose credentials include prior responsibility over one of the agencies charged with reviewing and clearing this drug for patient use. Upon closer examination, one finds that among the board members who will consider these issues over three years are those whose research findings Dr. Cooper's subordinate agency reviewed and to which he now refers as having proved the effective use of Valium.

Now, to complete the circle, a special consultant to this editorial board is the current administrator of the Alcohol, Drug Abuse, and Mental Health Administration at HEW, Dr. Gerald R. Klerman, previously a teaching professor at another well-known medical college. The series has been designed and funded, not by Cornell University, but by a company called Health Learning Systems, Inc., of which the chief operating officer is a former employee of Hoffman-LaRoche, the sponsoring company of research endeavors undertaken by several editorial board members and the producer of Valium, Librium, and Dalmane, the most widely prescribed tranquilizers in the world.

Only the clumsiness of the Hoffman-LaRoche Trojan Horse saved us from mass-media reports of predetermined "salutary findings." One of the reporter-employees that supply columnist Jack Anderson with many of his syndicated "inside stories" condemned this incestuous relationship in a recent Anderson column. Too often a muckraker, whose byline attracts attention, casts a pall on the integrity of his subject, warranted or not. At least in this case, it was helpful. But only for the moment have we been spared the inevitable campaign to improperly assign responsibility to the consumer for an imperfect — even injurious — product. The next attempt to enlarge the "ethical" pharmaceuticals' market is likely to be more subtle — and effective even now.

I am not a purist, nor a stoic. Scientific and technological progress is worth pursuing. Not only may life be extended, it can be enhanced. Human ingenuity must be encouraged — artistically, academically, or in commerce. But in our love affair with expanding knowledge, we must remember that every accomplishment, each creative endeavor, depends on the most extraordinary computer of all, the human brain. The complex system that the brain controls is the least understood. Yet we tinker with it thoughtlessly. Certainly, drug therapy has its place; but we have a right to know the price it may exact.

We even have the right to be made aware of uncertainty. The system of health care must be collaborative and we, the clients, ought to be included. When results affect personal health and behavior, it's unthinkable that others should be empowered to act without the subject's fully informed consent. It is required for surgery. It should be necessary for providing drugs that may alter basic functions. Perhaps if physicians and manufacturers were to be held accountable for untoward results, like addiction or other damage, such cautionary procedures would seem mutually agreeable. It's time to take stock. I don't believe that an increasingly concerned public will continue to accept the admonition *caveat emptor* as an appropriate canon of medical ethics.

In October 1978 representatives of the American Medical Association came before the House Select Committee on Narcotics Abuse and Control. In prepared testimony, Dr. Joseph Boyle said, "The general subject of the use and abuse of psychotrophic drugs is indeed a complex one. While there are national surveys that indicate how many prescriptions for a particular drug are written ... these surveys are not informative as to the many factors determining why a particular treatment regimen was ordered."

Another witness, Dr. Donald Rucker, professor at the College of Pharmacy of Ohio State University, said, "I am unaware of a single study in the literature able to document that prescriptions of psychoactive agents corresponded with standards of rational use established by the investigators." He added that reviews of specific studies related to the most popularly prescribed minor tranquilizers, Valium and Librium, showed that 75 percent of the prescriptions issued were for conditions inconsistent with the approved use for these drugs.

Perhaps that result is explained in another study by Ohio researchers. Sampled physicians were asked to identify the active chemical components in two commonly prescribed "combination" drugs, one of which was Librium. Only half of the doctors were able to answer correctly.

10

The Search for Help

MOST publicly funded treatment models — among them substitute-drug therapies and lifestyle modification techniques — have been designed to affect desirable change in the male body and in male behavior. The assumption on which they are based is simple and deadly: that drug addiction in our culture is primarily a male phenomenon. Until recent years, no special distinctions were made for females, and the results were appalling. Women who either voluntarily sought or were forced to seek help found themselves outnumbered, intimidated, and oppressed in largely male patient groups. Staffs were disproportionately male and were untrained in methods to accommodate rigid treatment patterns to the health and social needs of women clients. Only within this decade have the federal and state agencies for health begun to fund specific research, or collect data, on the service needs of women, needs that are often quite different from those of men.

The government's slow response is the result of several factors, not the least being an historic disinclination to tamper with society's expectations of perfection in womanhood. And most decision makers and highly funded researchers have been men whose sensitivity to differences between the sexes (except for reproductive functions) is minimal. Broadly speaking, this nation has been preoccupied with alcoholism and drug abuse as issues signifying violence, crime, and danger to persons and property.

There came the really troublesome point where the once neat distinction between legal and illegal drugs was muddied: *both* were associated with addiction. The greatest emerging problem among women seemed to implicate formidable industries and professions. Research, investigation, and attempts at treatment might be perceived as imputations of misfeasance or malpractice. This new dimension of political, legal, and economic trouble urged caution on all but the most courageous activists.

Inevitably it was in private sectors of the country, at community levels, where the human concern for health and function was first translated into action. Neighbors, families, and friends saw these drug invasions as cause more for empathy than fear. People-helping-people efforts were primarily responsible for the establishment of programs with better understanding of the diverse human condition, its strengths and weaknesses. Some of those nonbureaucratic commitments to human need have succeeded in gaining acceptance and even appropriations from governments for continued expansion of care.

Typically, women with drug- or alcohol-related problems instinctively seek advice from a physician, who unfortunately is the least likely source of effective care. Except in isolated cases, physicians are ill-equipped, and also disinclined, to treat or properly counsel addiction. Their lack of training and clinical experience, as well as their orientation to traditional chemical therapies for disease, accounts for their general inadequacy in this field. Many women have experienced embarrassment and disdain in the offices of inexpert, frustrated doctors. Even as they accept admonishment, they feel apologetic for discomfiting their physicians. Only an informed practitioner will be sensitive to the multifaceted nature of addictive diseases. Proper attention must be given to more than a single episode or symptom, and such attention may require the assistance of other care providers. The primary physician must be inclined to welcome collaboration, not feel threatened by it.

Hospital Treatment Programs

The comprehensive health care approach is gaining popularity among consumers and professionals alike. The expansion of general health-maintenance organizations confirms the effectiveness of whole-patient treatment either to treat chronic illness or to promote good health. This model is designed to provide a logical continuum of attention to all kinds of special needs. Its most salutary feature lies in the basic understanding that no single person or regimen may supply the full range of available wisdom or care.

This linkage approach may be the key to the successes of recently heralded drug treatment programs at facilities such as Long Beach Naval Hospital, where Betty Ford and Billy Carter were helped.

The Long Beach program has received so much publicity that there are now waiting lists for its magic. The formula that is employed in California is not a secret, however. Captain Joseph Pursch, USN, who directs that program, runs a spartan ship where well-known treatment elements are conscientiously applied. Dr. Pursch refers to many of his patients as "chemical gourmets," since often they have been heavy users of many legal drugs. The treatment model he uses is designed for the disease of alcoholism, but it seems to be effective for compulsive pill use as well. The patient's goal in treatment, Dr. Pursch declares, is to become a "recovering alcoholic." That label has the only status that counts at the center.

Although most patients arrive drug-free, there is a detoxification unit for those who need it. Thereafter, the routine appears deceptively simple, however complicated the addiction. Small therapy groups of seven to ten people spend three hours a day together. The groups meet morning and afternoon and are conducted by trained counselors who had been treated at the facility when they were enlisted personnel. During these sessions patients are prodded to discuss their alcoholism and to examine the likely reasons for their loss of control. Openness and candor are required. That sharing of common burdens becomes the foundation for mutual trust and supportive camaraderie. It is vital to successful integration into the larger fellowship of Alcoholics Anonymous meetings, which patients attend each evening. A daily group lecture, psychodrama sessions, regular work assignments, physical activity (jogging), and nutritious cafeteria meals punctuate the structured regimen.

After about three weeks, patients are generally given weekend passes and urged to test their new resolve by mingling with drinkers, at this halfway point in the program. When they return to the center they compare moods, feelings, and the challenges of coping. Occasionally, this review uncovers more severe, lingering problems. In those cases treatment may require eight or more weeks.

Whenever possible, certain group therapy sessions include husbands and wives of treatment patients. They become familiar with the spirit of the dialogue and by their presence, as well as new understanding, are able to give and receive acceptance as part of the caring team. A well-trained, dedicated staff leads addicted people through a process that is built on the philosophy that alcoholism is a treatable illness. But, unlike the medical germ-theory of disease, for which only chemicals and surgery are therapeutically imposed, this sickness is viewed within a social, biological complex. Thus the patient is involved in a process that defines illness, rebuilds health and function (preventive and curative), and interacts with nonmedical systems of care. A quite similar process is used at the nonmilitary Smithers Center at Roosevelt Hospital, New York, where Joan Kennedy seems to have fought her most successful battle against alcoholism.

Medical institutions with drug dependency components are increasingly available in public, private, and military settings. Although they have different criteria for admission and residential care, the programs in these institutions are usually based on this theory of continuity, beginning with medically supervised withdrawal from drugs. Depending on individual need and resources and the program's design, a patient may be in residence for two weeks or for months. Acute symptoms of addiction are reduced and healthy function is restored; nutritional and physical therapy is provided along with counseling. The primary objectives at this stage of rehabilitation are, first, an interpretation of drug use and, second, the introduction of alternative reinforcements for abstinent behavior. There are very practical reasons for seeking care in a medical unit within a larger hospital. Entrance into such a setting provides a degree of anonymity. Moreover, most health insurance policies provide for this type of care.

To assure long-term benefits, medical and other professional intervention techniques must soon be integrated with intermediate support programs outside the hospital environment. Adjunctive support groups serve an important function. They may be therapeutic community centers or mutual-aid associations. Some provide live-in, structured arrangements, others are social networks offering a community and language of common values. Whatever their dynamics, all attempt to redefine or renew the means and will for positive concepts and actions.

The Drug-Counseling Dilemma

Many public-health services are caught between separate funding authorities and are thus unable to provide needed services for certain drug-dysfunctional symptoms not deemed chronic diseases (diabetes, more than alcoholism, is considered chronic). I was told of a Chicago drug counselor's dilemma. A client who wanted to be humanely relieved of serious addictions to both opiates and alcohol was first put on a decreasing methadone therapy, only to be told later by the local hospitals that they would not treat for alcoholism while she was undergoing medical withdrawal from heroin. The counselor was caught in an administrative bind with a patient racing for survival. Fortunately, this caregiver decided to skirt the jurisdictional dictates and called upon compassionate colleagues to provide the necessary treatment.

Ironically, arbitrary discrimination still exists in some private groups and facilities as well. Although the reality of cross-addictions, particularly among women using legal drugs, has caused a gradual softening of rigid distinctions, bureaucratic elitism and contradiction must be taken into account in any search for help. Other factors to be considered in looking for help include the degree of medical supervision desirable for safe withdrawal, cost and location of the institution, and environment.

The sense of security that one environment may provide over another is often a decisive element. Many women prefer the private home settings of Women for Sobriety meetings over church or clubroom gatherings of Alcoholics Anonymous. These mutual-aid projects, although similar in a number of ways, have divergent policies that reflect and appeal to a diversity of people and kinds of problems and preferences. A setting in which an individual woman's differences and responses are understood and respected may certainly be the first step on the way to supportive friendship, thus hastening acceptance of self, others, and health.

Increasingly, benevolent coercion is being used to maneuver drug victims into counseling or medical treatment. This tactic has been used effectively by many industries and professional groups that have decided to admit the existence of a drug problem for some of their employees and have taken measures to alleviate it rather than continue to bear the enormous costs of concealment.

Enlightened management, often with the support of labor unions, has developed extensive "troubled employee" programs and policies. When job performance deteriorates, whether because of alcoholism, drug abuse, or emotional illness, treatment is offered as an alternative to dismissal or other sanctions.

Other groups as well have sought to disarm the problem and rehabilitate their members. In the military, the Navy network of services is notable. Problem drinking and drug use engendered great expense related to diseases, violence, and replacement of labor. Now live-in and nonresidential units of care process about 18,000 people yearly. In addition, an early screening and intervention safety program provides mandatory training and therapy for an estimated 11,000 men and women annually.

Addiction in the Helping Professions

The physician impaired by drugs or alcohol constitutes a serious hazard. Addictions among physicians have long been closely held, though not uncommon, secrets within the profession. Presently, more than half the states have passed legislation concerning sick doctors. An almost equal number of states have medical society service programs. Although the approach of each state or medical society may differ, the more effective impaired-physician programs can depend on active case finding, linkage with licensing boards, peer persuasion, and other methods to constrain on continued practice while the physician remains untreated. For obvious reasons, most of these efforts are kept strictly confidential and maintain a low profile. Men and women of the clergy have therapeutic retreats throughout the country, where faith and health are restored to the growing numbers who have succumbed to the contemporary malaise. Members of the religious community gather at North Conway Institute, in Massachusetts, each year for a three-day conference on their individual and collective responsibilities to minister to colleagues and congregants who have chemical dependencies. Last year I conducted a workshop on the special problems among women. Among the participants were a minister who identified herself as a recovered alcoholic and a priest with responsibility for several East Coast treatment centers for nuns.

In all these groups — corporate, military, professional, and religious — a therapeutic opportunity to continue to serve is provided by those who have the leverage of authority. However, studies document that compulsion *alone* seldom produces long-term abstinence. The programs accommodate that knowledge. The necessary hope and purpose that help defeat addiction are fostered by an atmosphere in which early detection and attention are followed by support and the reward of a viable career option. New survival skills offer the kind of bonus that many pension plans never considered.

There are many types of treatment models available for every type of dependency. In fact, certain helping techniques and programs that are useful for drug-dependent women are equally helpful to women who may never have had a drug problem. Assistance to health and fuller function is welcome and useful for all. Most women have some specific prior disability that needs to be overcome. Drugs may be only one factor impairing a fully functional life.

Some women's use of drugs is not so much dedicated as casual. By force of personal determination, many wean themselves from drug patterns. The catalyst to change differs. A new piece of information may trigger a personal challenge to be rid of the pattern. A friend's overdose or accident or a reported mishap may raise personal doubts and the realization that it might have been oneself. A newly found interest in health, recreation, or nutrition may vitalize self-concern. Some new purpose, environment, or awareness often promotes specific reassessment of old ways of feeling better; often it becomes a replacement that feels good. New options are taken every day, some before a drug-related crisis confounds the ability to make a willful change.

How to Recognize the Symptoms

There is no blanket set of symptoms to herald drug dependency to a casual observer. A truly dedicated user develops a sophisticated pattern of subterfuge, making identification of the problem difficult until an emergency occurs. In other cases, excuses for accidents or strange behavior are offered as the logical consequences of other coincidences. When assessing one's own vulnerability or that of another, unusual events must be viewed in the larger context of general condition, past and present. For example, one must ask whether the current aggressiveness, lassitude, insomnia, or lack of communication is a phase, a function of normal temperament, the occasional response to an identifiable problem, or a chronic, unusual, or unspecific condition. Habitual depression, slurred speech, frequent episodes of violent behavior, exaggerated mood-swings, and unsteady coordination may all be evidence of impairment. Whether or not they indicate drug taking or disease, they do signal distress and they require serious and immediate attention, communication, and advice.

Allowing for some exceptions, I do not agree with those who believe that a woman has to be on the skids before she will accept help. Even when acknowledgment of the problem is limited or efforts to change are only partially successful, each step is a positive alternative to an otherwise unbroken series of risks.

Lee's Story

Lee was doing part-time secretarial work when I met her. The first day she arrived at my office, she struggled through her typing chore, so critical of her own production that any frustration I felt paled by comparison. For stumbling through what she knew she could do better and faster, she insisted on an equitable reduction in hours charged to me. She was "feeling out of sorts" and would make up for it the next day, we agreed. For the next seven months, Lee worked diligently with me, as my small company designed, produced, and managed the first nationally held Forum on Drugs, Alcohol, and Women. It required intensive effort against many odds. There was so little time, funding, and commitment in 1975 to single out addicted women, and I insisted on an inclusive discussion, irrespective of existing emnity between the separate bureaucracies and specialists. Lee was stalwart. Her quirks were manifested in personal style, not in her dedication to the project or my purpose. I valued her innate qualities, her skills, resoluteness, and honesty. For some, her insistence on candor and whimsical mannerisms was confounding, especially since she appeared to have strong, practical reasoning power and abilities. The contrast troubled other staff members. I knew Lee was an unresolved young woman. Her outrageous, often earthy, pronouncements, her sudden decision to appear at the office dressed in a flimsy sari, her unsolicited details of some sexual adventure — all were expressions designed to shock, call attention to herself as "different," or to confirm her aliveness for herself.

During that year, technical literature dealing with the antisocial characteristics of drug-using young people described posturing like Lee's as "acting-out." Lee had problems, of that I was sure, although she kept her private space unavailable to real scrutiny. But she had value. I only invaded her intense world of quiet moods and tumultuous activity with the affection and trust I felt and expressed. When Lee left to take a legal assistant's job, we maintained only occasional contact. The full irony of her diligence in my employment has only recently become clear, in a letter she wrote me:

> I remember the first morning I came to work for you. I was so drunk from the night before, I could barely start the typewriter. And when I saw the project you were working on — well, all I could do was laugh.

That was in the late summer of 1975, and Lee was still taking diet pills (no longer effective in curbing her appetite), as she had been for the five previous years. She had begun looking for a womanly image right after completing high school. Make-up, high heels, older companions, and partying were her first expressions of "making it, on my own." But all those lunches out, dinners, and late-night dates added another dimension, excessive weight. As she wrote:

> My friend was putting on a little stomach too and she kept saying we had to locate this "fat doctor" she'd heard about. He was an internist downtown. I weighed in at 170 pounds. He put us on Delphetamine Stedytabs, gave us pep shots and B-12 injections. It gave me a terrific positive outlook,

lots of extra energy I'd never known, and I started dropping weight. For a few years, I went every week. I got my
shots and pills and wondered how I'd ever lived without
them. Whenever I took one it was like taking a miracle.

Lee loved the unbounded energy, available night or day,
feeling high, speeding along on her search for limitless experiences and confidence in herself. It was a way to ensure
that she wouldn't miss anything life had to offer. She remembered:

> Even if I had any bad times then, I would not have ascribed
> them to the pills. One time, I was visiting friends in Flor-
> ida. While they were at work, I took my pill and washed
> it down with a Coke. The next thing I knew, I'd defrosted
> the icy refrigerator. After my shower I decided that the
> shower curtain needed scrubbing and the bathroom needed
> redoing. I went to the five-and-dime store, bought the Con-
> Tact paper and redecorated the entire room. After that, I
> did an entire week's grocery shopping and made a month's
> worth of spaghetti sauce. Wasn't that good? (My friends
> thought so.) At least that's a good example of what speed's
> all about.

When the particular stimulant she had been ingesting was
taken off the market a few years later, Lee and her friend
were frantic. They went to every doctor and pharmacist
who might still have access to their favorite high. All they
could get was "a poor substitute." So to compensate, Lee took
two Tenuate Dospans at a time and worried constantly
about running out of her supply. "The thought was like
thinking of death." In fact, deathlike feelings were part of
the "depression that had been tearing me apart beginning
in the fall of 1973."

> By Christmas of 1974 I stopped smoking. I was a crying
> person. In February I gave notice at my job and after May
> did temporary work, slopped around a lot, increased my

drinking and lunching. I continued to take the pills, for energy, and ate anyhow. I was getting heavy again.

Her dates were patient with her constant bouts of depression; her friends enjoyed the continued drinking lunches. No one noticed trouble. Lee's pattern was altered, only for a while, by an event that caused fear and shame. She tried to piece it together, as follows:

I met a friend for lunch in my new white wool coat. I evidently left the bar, fell down on the way home, and was found by some ladies who knew me and the company that managed my apartment building. Somehow, they got me home. I must have been unconscious, because the next thing I remember was waking up in my smoke-filled apartment to answer a call from an out-of-town friend.

There was smoke everywhere and cooked hamburger all over the bed. Without that call, the apartment might have gone up in flames or I could have died from the smoke. My new white coat was filthy and I was scared. I couldn't face the resident manager and for a while lived with a lot of shame and less drinking. I only went overboard occasionally, after that.

Then Lee came to be needed, first by me, then by the man she plans to marry. Her needs changed. Her letter explains:

I threw away my pills that fall. I wanted to feel everything exactly as it was. It felt so good. I've found the meaning in my life. I can do just fine on my own, without the pills. I'm on the life track I'm supposed to be on. I've been able to put a lot into focus. I'm luckier than most and a lot stronger than I ever realized. Fortunately, I did what I did when I was young and got off while I was young enough to make substantial repairs. Not to mention that I found someone who cares.

The last line in her letter to me read: "I thought this would be a nice time to thank you for your friendship." She sent "much love" and a wedding invitation.

How much more could I have given to Lee? Shouldn't I have been more alert for symptoms? Perhaps. But Lee, like other bright individualists, learned how to parse out her relationships. She could perform a variety of discrete functions to meet the needs of others. She was adept at keeping her several worlds separate. Her privacy and pain were contained in prisons of her own keeping. Without access to more than a cubicle in another's life, insight, observation, and help are limited.

But love is not. And maybe, when you're very lucky, it's enough.

Awareness of the destructive consequences of continued drug use, while important, is only one of the ingredients of remedial action. The ability or willingness to institute a change depends on many things, including the duration of the dependency. The addicted person is often the one least able to see or control her destructive pattern. The chemical nature and subsequent effects of the drugs characteristically cause continued use; an alteration in body rhythms reinforces need, since discomfort is felt at the thought or fact of the drug's removal. There may even be a genuine incapacity to recall exact frequency of use or unpleasant events: memory functions may be drug-impaired. These behaviors must be understood to be a function of the chemicals, not judged as unhealthy choices or insincere responses to offers of help.

"If you think that just 'seeing the light' is the answer, you haven't asked the really hard questions." Lauren maintained that the real confrontation with a drug habit is only first met when one considers the alternative — life without it. "It's like agreeing to be deprived of your best friend, without being sure of whether you'll ever find another to rely on." Clearly, the decision to assist another person in breaking a long-established or intense relationship with drugs is a serious commitment. No less than with other life-saving strategies, successful intervention calls for knowledge of useful techniques, insight to common problems, understanding of any special circumstances, and, most importantly, unwavering support. Reliable comfort and belief, expressed by family, friends, or counselors, are strong influences. Dependency on drugs as surrogate friends may be reduced by the presence of new, human alternatives.

Different Treatments for Different People

A myriad of treatment philosophies have emerged in recent years and their differences are largely a matter of form and focus. All of them have a similar purpose, the reduction or elimination of chemical coping and disability. Conditions of personal need should dictate care, wherever possible. For example, if stigma is a sticking point, a community facility may be less appropriate, initially, than a more distant, less visible one. However, it should be understood that all health records and procedures are strictly confidential and personnel are extremely sensitive to privacy needs. Still, some women are disinclined to participate in helping groups of any kind, preferring instead to see trained professionals in private practice or to associate with outpatient hospital or clinic centers.

No single approach is equally effective for every woman. Some women do not require any of the traditionally described programs. A talking therapy and camaraderie may be better found at a women's center in a local university or college. The result of private assessment may point the way to career guidance as a strategy for new direction and growth. Many community organizations and colleges provide new-skills courses, assertiveness classes, reality therapy training, continuing education programs. They also offer new collegial networks.

Any of these groups may supply a most important non-chemical medication, even for those who eventually question the continuing value of the group. That medication is the tincture of time that allows distance from drugs, making change possible.

The Alcoholics Anonymous movement is considered the paradigm for most self-help groups. These organizations have common characteristics. They are voluntary groups whose members share similar problems or handicaps. They meet on a regular basis to express their experiences and efforts for change. They support each other with skills, concern, and knowledge through personal interaction. Through this affiliation, common bonds are forged. Eventually, those who come to be helped are helped most by providing assistance to others. The very process of exchange, deemed valuable by the members, enhances individual self-esteem and social usefulness. Through codified language techniques, role models, and ritual procedures, each group establishes separate, loyal memberships.

In recent years these previously traditional units have been altered by the presence of increasing numbers of women. Some have formed all-women groups, or separate sex counseling; others have added child-care or family components, all in response to better meeting female requirements. The therapeutic value of many self-help groups is a source of primary treatment for many women who may not require a medical setting. Whether a woman elects residential care or outpatient family or individual therapy, the ongoing support and growth fostered by these special purpose groups can add a new dimension of assistance.

Increasing numbers and types of helping services for women are now being established throughout the country. Although certain of them focus on the particular problems associated with drug or alcohol addiction, others encompass a broader range of crisis intervention, referral, or emergency shelter. Without knowledge of the special emphasis of these group activities, or even awareness of the availability of support efforts, many women are denied acceptable assistance.

The predominant technique in male-oriented treatment settings is confrontation. Challenging the patient's perceptions of self-sufficiency and power rights, the process of restoring functional equilibrium depends on knocking out the props that sustain notions of supremacy. Beyond merely challenging the defiant use of drugs as an exercise in personal choice, the staff embarks on a systematic effort to alter the "macho" facade. Values are ridiculed. Strengths are questioned as being no more than compensation for pitiable weakness. In some instances, humility is imposed by such visible embarrassments as head-shaving or having to wear self-deprecating signs. Admissions of personal need are viewed as signs of growth and rehabilitation.

Obviously this routine works for some, even for some women whose survival necessitated an appearance of indomitable strength and independence. But this approach is terribly destructive to others, particularly to many females. If a woman's reliance on drugs stems from her lack of belief in herself, her anxiety about the judgment of others, or the absence of a reliable network of friends, then a therapy that reinforces her deficits is inimical to redressing her wounds.

For most women, an encounter with the truth of willful or accidental addiction must be woven through a fabric of support and encouragement. Recognition of destructive behavior should enhance, not debilitate, personal striving for healthy self-determination.

The changes adopted by programs that reach out to women in need embrace a spectrum of issues that are understood to effect the real concerns of those who might otherwise remain hidden or unidentified.

Even in those places where both sexes are treated, women professionals are available to provide leadership and counseling. Women-only groups are held to allow for uninhibited discussions of sexuality, troubling family dynamics, responsibilities of motherhood, or the burdens of physical discomfort and unfulfilled dreams.

Because of the continuing social stigma against anything perceived as deviant or abnormal, some programs are deliberately undesignated as therapeutic projects and operate as informal centers for social activities and skills development. However, these community centers often combine yoga with self-awareness, they offer parent-effectiveness training, gynecological examinations, and have groups in which women can share experiences and explore the limitations caused by stereotyping. Frequently, "rap sessions" become mutual-aid, "old-girl networks."

Most notable women's programs are designed to accommodate work and family responsibilities and make arrangements for child care.

For women, the process of reconstructing emotional and physical health must put the negative event of addiction into its limited and limiting context. Seen as a problem resulting from one of many influences, not the centerpiece of inherent character pathology, addiction can be treated by diminishing the causes in part by building skills, will, and trust. Self-control is urged and supported by gentle guidance and acceptance. A positive emphasis is placed on individual awareness and potential growth. Friendship is fostered, as are healthy relationships in other spheres of life. Long-term dependency is discouraged, whether it be on staff members and group wisdom or on others for personal truths or values. Professionals with a feminist orientation believe that the most difficult battle for women is the one between conditioned acquiescence and learning the ability to make their own choices.

At the end of this book is a selectively compiled listing of state offices and agencies responsible for supplying drug and alcohol information and services. A brief directory of medical or counseling centers and national self-help organizations with local chapters is also provided to supplement listings that may be found in local telephone directories.

The diversity of existing projects is considerable, as the following thumb-nail sketches indicate.

Today, Inc., is located in Newton, Pennsylvania. Designed for young adults, this therapeutic community treats male and female multidrug abusers as residents and outpatients, using methods that employ separate and mixed-sex groups.

In Los Angeles, The Institute for Studies of Destructive Behavior and the Suicide Prevention Center houses a family development program. Group, individual, and family counseling are offered to pregnant women, parents, and preschool children. Day care facilities are provided, and psychological testing and education in child development are given, as well as referrals for medical and legal aid.

At the Medical College of Virginia Hospital, in Charlottesville, the Adolescent Medicine Clinic provides detoxification, one-to-one counseling, and medical attention to gynecological problems. Group therapy is available, as are classes in self-defense, rape prevention, contraception, and self-awareness.

Women Together is a state-funded outpatient program in Glassboro, New Jersey, for women who are dependent on legal drugs. The corollary is a twenty-four-hour hotline (Together, Inc.) that offers assistance in any crisis as well as information and referral.

Meta House, in Milwaukee, is a women-only live-in treatment facility. Located in a residential neighborhood, it's a gentle setting for the careful restructuring of an alcohol- or drug-ridden life. The treatment process, which includes part-time or full-time work outside the halfway house, takes from thirty to ninety days.

At Eagleville Hospital, just outside Philadelphia, Family House is a rehabilitation center for mothers with young children. While their children's care is attended to, residents spend from six months to a year learning to live without their addictions, which frequently include both drugs and alcohol. Simultaneously, they are provided with job skills, parenting insight, and stronger self-concepts.

Community Crisis Center, Inc., is a multiservice program for women in Elgin, Illinois. Shelter is available if needed. The center is a source of referral to needed care. It offers counseling by telephone or in person, as the client prefers, and is open twenty-four hours a day, daily.

Transition House, located at the Women's Center in Cambridge, Massachusetts, holds weekly support-group meetings. Through an all-day and all-night hotline other crises are handled quickly, including referrals to proper social, legal, and medical assistance. The resident shelter for women and children victimized by violence provides legal advocates to assure protection. This facility is also a training ground for volunteers who wish to become legal advocates.

Alternatives to drug use are taught at the Janus Growth Center in Baltimore. During a twelve-week group therapy course, clients are led through sessions including meditation, yoga, psychodrama, dance, music, and art. Whole-person health is emphasized. Only some of the participants have personal histories of drug use.

There is an outstanding program in Minneapolis, Minnesota. For years it has been the center of a full range of services for women. Its dedicated staff provides counseling and guidance on legal, vocational, social, and behavioral issues. It has become a meeting place for many women, only some with problems of addiction. The name of the program is Chrysalis, a word that defines the golden sheath from which a butterfly emerges.

Help does exist. And by whatever crucible, each woman may find her chrysalis.

11

Finding Yourself Without Drugs

H. L. MENCKEN once said, "There is a solution to every problem — quick, simple, and wrong."

There is no single female experience. A search for insight into what it means to be female must consider the variables; individual behavior seldom occurs in a vacuum. Culture, age, and personal values are all part of a constellation of factors to be examined. If women have unique characteristics, they also face differing options and resources. Even when mindful of the self-deprecating feelings and the life stresses that may precipitate a turn to chemical solutions, one must have both will and the skills with which to identify susceptibility. Time, energy, and encouragement are also required to resolve or modify the condition. Except in laboratory settings, most people act on feelings and beliefs, not reason alone.

I have often sat with colleagues exploring coincidences or perceptions affecting human endeavor. The search for some universal laws — even straws — proves elusive. Always we could agree on the obvious dynamics leading to ritual drug or alcohol use. We understood the phenomenon of loneliness that accompanies legal addictions. We were familiar with many of the helping techniques that have greater or lesser success among women, some quite different from those applied to men. But, what about common clues?

During a recent discussion, we focused on whether the act of conferring complete faith in a supreme destiny was an abdication of responsibility or an element of mature strength. Patty wondered if some equation could be drawn from a willingness to believe in intangibles, external to yourself, that would "take care of you." Is that a transferable mind set? Could power then be bestowed on various masters, whether these were fate, bourbon, or Dalmane? She recalled a friend who, during the four years of intensive drug taking, came to believe that everything that felt good was made possible by the drugs she was using, and likewise anything that went badly could be remedied by taking a drug.

> She never believed that anything would happen purely as a result of her actions, her own contribution. Janet didn't make things happen — the pills did. Amphetamines were the source of her creative energy. Tranquilizers were the source of her gentleness. On the other hand, the drugs afforded her an excuse for her actions when she needed it. Eventually she came to know that they also denied her any personal "ownership" of her accomplishments or pleasures.

Ellen recalled a close friend who, as a young adult, cast off orthodox Roman Catholicism and became antagonistic to all formal religion. In later years, because of a problem with alcohol, this friend became very active in Alcoholics Anonymous, an organization with a strong spiritual base. She did not find her commitment to AA incompatible with her dissociation from formal religion. She explained to Ellen:

> AA allowed me a personal definition of a superior power. I can accept that. It frees me to acknowledge the limitations of my humanity; to understand that most people's reach exceeds their grasp. That approach permits me to

admit my need for outside strength, but it goes further. In this supporting environment, I am not made to feel defensive about weakness. In fact, I'm urged to reach for my own special strength. It's comforting to know, by the examples of others, that you may not be able to do it alone, but only you can do it.

Many successful mutual-help groups have effectively communicated the need for a balanced perspective on inside strengths and outside forces. Theories of what is possible are translated into measurable personal actions. Each successful result, however small, promotes further purposeful efforts. Rewarded by others' interest and positive regard, self-esteem and strength of purpose are serenely enhanced.

The universal scheme of things produces different responses. For some it is so awesome that peace is only possible by acquiescing and assigning all responsibility for times and tides to something other than one's frail self. In recent times we have witnessed how this submissive posture has been put to destructive use by cult leaders. In all of human history, institutionalized surrender has been the hallmark of fanatic, inhuman eras and events. It diminishes individual significance and possibility, producing a vacuum easily filled by dogma bearing good or evil purpose. The same result is possible for those who are so narcissistic that the dimension and quality of their lives are limited by their completely disallowing that factors outside themselves should have any effect on personal pursuits. Pleasure and pain alike have only transitory or hollow meaning for such people.

Somewhere between total surrender and presumptuous arrogance is a reasoned, responsible understanding of the promise and the process of which we are each a part. But we must each assess elements of conditioning, be willing to confront reality, and invest in our own destiny.

My friend Ellen insists that particular life roles are so ingrained in the female personality that many women are not even aware of their conditioned responses. To illustrate the point, she reminded me of the perceptive observation that Jane O'Reilly had made and then written about in a column for *The Washington Star*. She recalled a day when, in a supermarket, she accidentally bumped into another woman customer with her food cart. Before O'Reilly could apologize to the innocent bystander, the victim smiled, retreated, and said, "I'm so sorry." Perplexed, the writer decided to find out whether that was an isolated reaction or a patterned response. She proceeded deliberately to run her cart into ten other blameless women. Each offered an undeserved apology. In reflecting on this event, O'Reilly became aware of the many times she had apologized for things she could not control. She recognized how commonplace it is to hear women apologize, about everything. Ellen paraphrased the article's observations of some typical excuses:

> Sorry the weather isn't working out; I'm sorry you had a bad day; sorry you fell and bumped your head; sorry you hate your job; sorry that the roads are bad, that the snow is falling, and just when you were coming for the weekend.

"You see," Ellen continued, "some selfless behavior is mindless. Constant nurturing and dependence on approval create a model attitude for other compulsive habits. A woman who subliminally feels responsible for making everything perfect can't possibly live up to that expectation. She exhausts herself trying or just retreats."

Where does one find the common denominator most likely to shake out the unseen or denied dependency and convert it into "I can't live this way anymore, I want to be alive"? The search for that survival piece of the puzzle has been intense but unyielding of absolutes. Before reaching a point of readiness to undo a habit, however unhealthy, a woman has to meet at least two other conditions. The first is a willingness to recognize the existence of the pattern. The other is the courage to question the validity of oft-used personal ploys and rationalizations for drug use.

For example, at a meeting with several rehabilitative health specialists recently, two troubling incidents were described. Helen had a visit with an old school friend whom she had not seen in many years. She notes,

> I was appalled. Each night she had an hour-long ritual to prepare for sleep. She took three or four different pills, carefully arranged the drapes to assure no distractions of light, checked the air flow in her room, and put on her eye shades. She attended to all of these things ritualistically. When I described my work with women and addictions, deliberately drawing out the discussion about compulsive behavior, she was fascinated but remained personally aloof. She couldn't identify with that at all.

Peggy told about a relative.

> In addition to seeing her pop pills morning and evening, I noticed her hitting the bar. I commented that I didn't know she liked to drink. She replied, "I didn't know it either. I do know that I was becoming impossible to live with. I snapped at everyone. I was worried and tense all the time — they told me so. So, I figured it out. All of this stuff makes me a nicer person. Everyone thinks so. You might call it my niceness diet. It's better than being the way I was before."

When a woman with a chemical compulsion is ready neither to see nor characterize it, she may for as many reasons deny it. Depression, anxiety, and drug use all have a core of compromise with deep-seated emotional conflict. Denial is a logical response. So long as a woman is unwilling or unable to confront what her drug use has buried, her survival defense will firmly refute her recognition that she is dependent on drugs. Even private acknowledgment of the mask would not necessarily lead to removing it, for drugs are knowingly employed as an acceptable, partial solution to painful, unacceptable, or immutable conditions. Without known alternatives, a tradeoff may be more terrifying. It is easy to be confused by the sharp, yet finely imperceptible, line of distinction between the behavior of those who are coping, in strength, and that of those who are captives, in weakened submission. With drugs the line will eventually be crossed. Then a major life crisis may surface — and that is the cutting edge.

Over the years, I've known personally and heard of many women who either considered or committed suicide. Some of these women used drugs as their active weapon against the world and themselves. Others, whose addictive personalities and lives were painfully empty, accepted drugs passively, thus acceding to complete victimization. Setting aside those instances where a degenerative or other disease was the primary rationale for drug-induced suicide attempts, I've tried to search out some critical differences between those who succumbed and those who survived.

I've known women who have scrupulously planned detailed scenarios of their own death (even including "doing two weeks' laundry for the children"), but who have stopped short at the end and said, "I can't do that." Others have recounted occasions when "It seemed the only thing to do. I'll never understand why I didn't do it." I reviewed these cases, looking for some link. All I could find in common, at first, was despair and fatigue. But after sifting further through all of their expressions of alarm, reflective horror, and persistent wonderment, I discovered something else. Without exception each of the survivors overcame the final crisis with a grasp (often more tentative than firm) of her personal life journey and a connected purpose. In many cases, mundane events would provide signals of her worth — that she was needed by one or more people. It made all the difference, that she made a difference!

At that moment of recognition — unastonishing at the time and even later remaining an indiscernible event — each of them saw and chose life as more meaningful than the alternative. What is more important is that by her inaction she makes a choice. For some, the event of selection itself is momentous. It signifies, in tangible terms, that they — on their own terms — can make a crucial decision.

Those who succumbed to defeat were in almost every case living in a scenario designed and written by others. Their lives had been lived by rote, eroded by time and by the rough edges of external circumstances. These women had depended overwhelmingly on forces outside themselves to give their lives meaning. They had no faith in their own, independent value, or they placed no value in faith. They had no immediate or universal strengths to draw upon. No overriding raison d'être. There were no small voices to say, "You have made a difference; you can make a difference; what you are and what you do makes a difference."

How does one convey to another or believe for oneself that each of us counts for something worthwhile and that each day brings new and valuable possibilities? We can help those we love learn to value themselves. It's never too late. It just takes more convincing, the later it begins.

Over the years of confronting the challenges and decisions in my own life, I have grown ever more grateful for my grandparents' influence. Throughout their daily lives, they loved me, unqualifiedly, sufficiently to have caused me to be sure that I was "special." Among my earliest recollections are their loving reminders of my inheritance — thousands of years of recorded history and ancestors. Considering oneself the child of a chosen people sorely tried by an exacting Creator might have had terrifying implications, but my grandparents chose to interpret traditional responsibilities as but one aspect of their cultural legacy. I was instructed that all traditions and rituals are subject to personal interpretation and definition. In fact, they made it emphatic that questioning, analyzing, and accepting or rejecting — even sacred commentaries — were basic rights and requirements of our heritage. What they imparted to me became the core of my personal strength.

There are, I learned, no automatic, thoughtless answers, no intermediaries to accept responsibility for one's acts. The righteous life my grandparents described requires each person to use fully whatever talents, wisdom, kindness, and strengths he or she possesses. No one else's measure of best or proper is necessarily more appropriate than one's own. Each has the right and the duty to question, to choose, to act. Each is expected to justify or remedy the results of individual actions, using reason and heart. Mistakes are not only tolerated, they are corrected and learned from — reconstructing them attests to greater human possibilities.

I was provided with the past, as a touchstone, the present as an extension of the ongoing experiment, and the future as a place of potential that invited my own distinctive style. I have been lucky. When confronted by folly, uncertainty, unfairness, or grief, I have drawn will and purpose from a reservoir of redeemable promise. But my strength is essentially the past memory of childhood; I must renew it by acting it out. Only by redesign and redefinition, to meet the challenge of the dilemmas I encounter, do I revitalize my own belief in personal capacity. So must we all.

Obviously my convictions are tempered by experience. I have been close to many women who have overcome traumatic events, some precipitated by drugs. One said, confirming my view,

> I don't know why we have to take so long, acting like a piece of clay . . . all the while we pretend to be invincible. None of that is really true. I had to go through that awful chemical cop-out, which almost did me in, before I realized the truth of myself. The surest way to feel like a misfit

and in constant fear is to spend all your energy trying to "fit in." People don't fit neatly into the same boxes.

Another said,

> I still maintain there is a need for faith in yourself. I went to a psychiatrist for a long time. I knew I was losing touch with reality after all the pills and booze. I tried to get everything back together again. I pretended it was helping. It wasn't. The change doesn't really happen until it happens in yourself . . . how you feel about yourself.

These women, like most of us, had to sort out many things in order to find themselves. They had to scrutinize intensely themselves and those they loved. They had to learn that self-destructive patterns are controllable, that a new perspective on old myths is both necessary and possible. They had to practice the introspection and acquire the information that are requisite in defeating exploitative behaviors. They had to ask the questions: What are my strengths? What would I change? Can I? How? Will that affect my self-assurance? Will a better me please those who matter to me? Will I like a less dependent, more dependable me? Am I willing to undergo some period of discomfort to become more of the best of me? Each of us must wonder: By short-circuiting my body's own ability to provide its own remedy, am I inviting some parts to function less well or to atrophy from disuse?

The human quest to exceed the limited expectations of unexplored ability is endangered by mood merchants who freely bombard us with immediate and narrowing solutions. (As Mencken said: "simple and wrong.") In the face of this, we must remain energetic in pursuit of the phenomenon of our humanity.

We must hold dear our capacity to feel, think, and choose. If we do — and only if we do — what looks and feels like a stumbling block may yet become a steppingstone. Personal choice, not magic, makes all things possible.

Women cannot wait for institutions to reform. Each of us pursuing a rightful, shared responsibility for personal health must demand better information and a more responsive, responsible system of care. We must act as though our lives depend on our insights and decisions. They do.

If history is prologue, then we must learn that separately and in groups we form generations and constitute the future. We must defy a cruel conformity to a hopeless, drugged past in order to nourish a kinder legacy. Our responsibility to ourselves and to life's potential must begin where all hope begins — in individuals, in ourselves.

Appendix: Where to Find Help

In order to encourage women to make active choices, a range of options must be made available to them. During this past decade, or longer, hundreds of theoretical and technical approaches to chemical dependency and compulsive behaviors have been espoused. Some are being employed by formal programs of treatment and rehabilitation; others by the burgeoning number of self-help, less formalized groups throughout the country.

In this section, I offer the names and addresses of various programs, agencies, and centers throughout the country, to enable a first step toward health. The information may be more than some want, less than others need. But it is a beginning, offered in friendship and hope.

State Programs

EVERY STATE AND TERRITORY of the United States that receives health funds from the federal government administers them under the auspices of an acceptable state or territorial agency or department. In most jurisdictions a separate division is assigned to have authority over the dissemination of moneys and materials related to drug and alcohol problems.

Since 1976, after Congressmen Peter W. Rodino, Jr. (D–N.J.) and Paul Rogers (D–Fla.), along with Senators William Hathaway (D–Maine) and Harrison Williams (D–N.J.), successfully amended existing legislation, programs of assistance to women have been required in each state. Some states have been more diligent than others.

Nonetheless, as official arms of the Department of Health, Education, and Welfare, state offices are the repositories of both local and national information on available services, research findings, and organizational philosophies relating to all aspects of crisis and chronic health-care issues. Each citizen's request for general or specific inquiry should be honored, willingly.

Since 1978, many new projects have been initiated for women. That pattern should continue. To assure that any question of state law regarding insurance, parental rights, or any other civil rights may be answered — thus reducing inhibitions to seek effective treatment — the state office (provided in the following list) should be called. Additionally, these offices may provide current listings of public and private programs.

Alabama

Alcoholism and Drug Abuse
  Division
Department of Mental Health
502 Washington Ave.
Montgomery, AL 36130
(205) 265-2301

Alaska

Department of Health and Social
  Services
Office of Alcoholism and Drug
  Abuse
Pouch H-05F
Juneau, AK 99811
(907) 586-3585
(Seattle FTS Operator 8-399-0150)

Arizona

Chief, Bureau of Program Operations
Division of Behavioral Health
  Services
2500 E. Van Buren St.
Phoenix, AZ 85008
(602) 255-1229

Arkansas

Director
Office of Alcohol and Drug Abuse
  Prevention
1515 W. 7th St.
Little Rock, AR 72202
(501) 371-2604

California

Department of Alcohol and Drug
  Abuse
825 15th St.
Sacramento, CA 95814
(916) 322-6690

Colorado

Alcohol and Drug Abuse Division
Department of Health
4210 E. 11th Ave.
Denver, CO 80220
(303) 320-1167

Connecticut

Executive Director
Alcohol and Drug Abuse Council
90 Washington St.
Hartford, CT 06115
(203) 566-4145

Delaware

Bureau of Substance Abuse
Division of Mental Health
1901 North du Pont Highway
New Castle, DE 19720
(302) 421-6101

District of Columbia

Assistant Director
Department of Human Resources
1329 "E" St., N.W.
Washington, D.C. 20004
(202) 724-5696

Florida

Drug Abuse Program
Mental Health Program Office
1317 Winewood Blvd.
Tallahassee, FL 32304
(904) 488-0900

Georgia

Division of Mental Health and
  Retardation
Georgia Department of Human
  Resources
618 Ponce de Leon Ave., N.E.
Atlanta, GA 30308
(404) 894-4785

Hawaii

State Substance Abuse Agency
1270 Queen Emma St.
Honolulu, HI 96813
(808) 548-7655

Idaho

Bureau of Substance Abuse
State House
700 W. State St.
Boise, ID 83720
(208) 384-3920

Illinois

Executive Director
Illinois Dangerous Drugs Commission
300 N. State St.
Chicago, IL 60610
(312) 822-9860

Indiana

Division of Addiction Services
5 Indiana Sq.
Indianapolis, IN 46204
(317) 633-4477

Iowa

Department of Substance Abuse
Suite 230, Liberty Building
418 6th Ave.
Des Moines, IA 50319
(515) 281-3641

Kansas

Alcohol and Drug Abuse Section
Biddle Building
Topeka State Hospital
2700 W. 6th St.
Topeka, KS 66606
(913) 296-3925

Kentucky

Department of Human Resources
Bureau for Health Services
275 E. Main St.
Frankfort, KY 40601
(502) 564-7610

Louisiana

Office of Hospitals
200 Lafayette St.
Baton Rouge, LA 70804
(504) 342-2575

Maine

Office of Alcohol and Drug
  Abuse
Department of Human Services
32 Winthrop St.
Augusta, ME 04330
(207) 289-2781

Maryland

Drug Abuse Administration
201 W. Preston St.
Baltimore, MD 20201
(301) 383-3959

Massachusetts

Division of Drug Rehabilitation
Department of Mental Health
160 N. Washington St.
Boston, MA 02114
(617) 727-8614

Michigan

Office of Substance Abuse
  Services
3500 N. Logan St.
Lansing, MI 48909
(517) 373-8600

Minnesota

Chemical Dependency — DPW
Centennial Office Building
658 Cedar, 4th Floor
St. Paul, MN 55155
(612) 296-4610

Mississippi

Division of Alcohol and Drug
  Abuse
619 Robert E. Lee Office Building
Jackson, MS 39201
(601) 354-7031

Missouri

Department of Mental Health
2002 Missouri Blvd.
Jefferson City, MO 65101
(314) 751-4942

Montana

Alcohol and Drug Division
Department of Institutions
1539 11th Ave.
Helena, MT 59601
(406) 449-2827

Nebraska
Nebraska Commission on Drugs
Box 94726
Lincoln, NE 68509
(402) 471-2691

Nevada
Bureau of Alcohol and Drug
  Abuse
505 King St.
Carson City, NV 89710
(702) 885-4790

New Hampshire
Office of Drug Abuse Prevention
3 Capitol St., Rm. 405
Concord, NH 03301
(603) 271-2754

New Jersey
Alcohol, Narcotic and Drug
  Abuse
Department of Health
129 E. Hanover St.
Trenton, NJ 08608
(609) 292-5760

New Mexico
Substance Abuse Bureau
Behavioral Health Services
Health and Environmental
  Department
Box 968
Santa Fe, NM 87503
(505) 827-5271

New York
Division of Substance Abuse
  Services
Executive Park South
Albany, NY 12203
(518) 457-2061

North Carolina
Alcohol and Drug Abuse
325 N. Salisbury St.
Raleigh, NC 27611
(919) 733-4555

North Dakota
Division of Alcoholism and Drug
  Abuse
Mental Health and Retardation
  Services
909 Basin Ave.
Bismarck, ND 58505
(701) 224-2767

Ohio
Bureau of Drug Abuse
State Office Tower, Rm. 1352
30 E. Broad St.
Columbus, OH 43215
(614) 466-7604

Oklahoma
Drug Abuse Services
Box 53277
Oklahoma City, OK 73105
(405) 521-2811

Oregon
Mental Health Division
2575 Bittern St., N.E.
Salem, OR 97310
(503) 378-2163

Pennsylvania
Governor's Council on Drug and
  Alcohol Abuse
2101 N. Front St.
Harrisburg, PA 17120
(717) 787-9857

Rhode Island
Division of Substance Abuse
Building 303, General Hospital
Rhode Island Medical Center
Cranston, RI 02920
(401) 464-2091

South Carolina
South Carolina Commission on
  Alcohol and Drug Abuse
3700 Forest Dr.
Columbia, SC 29204
(803) 758-2183

South Dakota

Division of Drugs and Substances
  Control
Department of Health
Joe Foss Building
Pierre, SD 57501
(605) 773-3123

Tennessee

Alcohol and Drug Abuse Services
  Section
501 Union Building
Nashville, TN 37219
(615) 741-1921

Texas

Drug Abuse Prevention Division
Department of Community
  Affairs
210 Barton Springs Rd.
Austin, Texas 78704
(512) 475-5566

Utah

Division of Alcohol and Drugs
150 W. North Temple
Rm. 350
Salt Lake City, UT 84110
(801) 533-6532

Vermont

Alcohol and Drug Abuse Division
Agency of Human Services
State Office Building
Montpelier, VT 05602
(802) 241-2170

Virginia

Department of Mental Health
  and Mental Retardation
Box 1797
Richmond, VA 23214
(804) 786-5313

Washington

Department of Social and Health
  Services
OB-43E
Olympia, WA 98504
(206) 753-3073

West Virginia

Alcohol and Drug Abuse Program
State Capitol
Charleston, WV 25305
(304) 348-3616

Wisconsin

Bureau of Alcohol and Drug
  Abuse
1 W. Wilson St.
Madison, WI 53702
(608) 266-2717

Wyoming

Mental Health and Mental
  Retardation Services
Hathaway Building, Rm. 451
Cheyenne, WY 82002
(307) 777-7115

Puerto Rico

Department of Addiction Control
  Services
Box B-Y
Rio Piedras Station
Rio Piedras, PR 00928
(809) 763-8957 or 763-7575

Pacific Trust Territories

Division of Mental Health
Department of Health Services
Office of the High Commissioner
Saipan, Mariana Islands 96950

Guam

Mental Health and Substance
  Abuse Health Agency
Box 20999
Guam, Mariana Islands 96921

Virgin Islands

Division of Mental Health, Alco-
  holism and Drug Dependency
Box 520
Christiansted
St. Croix, VI 00820
(809) 774-4888 or 249-7959

Treatment Resources

To OBTAIN specific treatment or referral information, as well as advice on available care, costs, and methods, you must make inquiries and decisions. The following list of programs and institutions has been culled from more extensive listings compiled by the National Institute on Drug Abuse and the National Institute on Alcohol Abuse and Alcoholism and from various state and private documents. Although several references for each state are given, many more exist.

Some programs of help are designed for certain selected populations. Among the matters you should discuss with a representative of any program, in person or by telephone, are your age, economic status, and the nature of your health problems, as well as whether you require single or co-sex facilities and resident or outpatient care. If your criteria for comfort are not met at one facility, another should be sought. Openly indicate your preferences, concerns, and needs. Although I cannot personally assess each of the programs listed here, I can say that they are designated as treatment or service resources by federal, state, and private sources. They were established to provide assistance and are anxious to do so.

Alabama
Eastside Mental Health Center
Birmingham, AL 35205
(205) 833-3460

Salvation Army Girls Lodge
1509 12th Ave. South
Birmingham, AL 35205
(205) 933-0717

University of Alabama
  Birmingham Hospital
1919 7th Ave. South
Birmingham, AL 35233
(205) 934-5164

St. Anne's Home, Inc.
2772 Hanover Circle
Birmingham, AL 35205
(205) 933-6906

Tranquilaire Hospital
251 Cox St.
Mobile, AL 36604
(205) 432-8811

Greil Hospital
2140 Upper Wetumpka Rd.
Montgomery, AL 36107

Alaska
The Family Rap
2825 W. 42nd Pl.
Anchorage, AK 99503
(907) 279-5502

Island Counseling Center
543 8th Ave.
Fairbanks, AK 99701
(907) 452-1841

Nome Walk In Center
Nome, AK 99762
(907) 279-1408

Arctic Cache
Box 933
North Pole, AK 99705
(907) 488-2222

Arizona
Behavioral Health Agency of
  Central Arizona
102 N. Florence St.
Casa Grande, AZ 85222
(602) 836-1688

Pinal Alcohol/Drug Addiction
  Council Mt. Drug Prevention
  Center

111 W. First St.
Casa Grande, AZ 85222
(602) 836-0648

Camelback Hospital
5055 N. 34th St.
Phoenix, AZ 85018
(602) 955-6200

Community Behavioral Services
700 W. Campbell St.
Phoenix, AZ 85013
(602) 264-2341

Maricopa County General
  Hospital
Psychiatric Unit
2601 E. Roosevelt
Phoenix, AZ 85008
(602) 267-5011

North Mountain Behavioral
  Institute
2836 E. Van Buren St.
Phoenix, AZ 85008
(602) 944-4641

St. Joseph's Hospital and Medical
  Center
350 W. Thomas Rd.
Phoenix, AZ 85013
(602) 277-6611

Apache County Guidance Clinic
Fran Whiting Memorial Hospital
St. Johns, AZ 85936
(602) 337-4301

Tri-City Mental Health Center
Full Circle
424 W. Broadway
Tempe, AZ 85285
(602) 967-8586

Amity House
9560 E. Old Spanish Trail
Tucson, AZ 85710
(602) 886-5557

Palo Verde Hospital
801 S. Prudence Rd.
Tucson, AZ 85710
(602) 298-3363

The Haven
1107 E. Adelaide
Tucson, AZ 85719
(602) 623-4590

The Foundation of Arizona, Inc.
1050 N. Cherry
Tucson, AZ 85712
(602) 327-1734

Awareness House of Yuma
712 S. 2nd Ave.
Yuma, AZ 85364
(602) 783-5411

Catholic Social Services
2450 S. 4th Ave.
Yuma, AZ 85364
(602) 344-2840

Arkansas
North Central Arkansas Mental
  Health Center
Highway 25 North
Batesville, AR 72501
(501) 268-2449 or 793-6383

Ozark Guidance Center
Bentonville Center
Bentonville, AR 72712
(501) 273-2113

Human Services Center of West
  Central Arkansas
1622 N. Donagney
Conway, AR 72032
(501) 327-7706 or 329-2989

Western Arkansas Counseling
  and Guidance Center
910 S. 12th St.
Fort Smith, AR 72901
(501) 452-6650

Mid-Delta Community Services,
  Inc.
Alcoholism Program
622 Pecan St.
Helena, AR 72342
(501) 338-6408

Arkansas Mental Health Services
4313 Markham St.
Little Rock, AR 72203
(501) 666-0181

Ozark Regional Mental Health
  Center
Mountain Home Clinic
Mountain Home, AR 72653
(501) 425-6439

Family Service Agency of Pulaski
  County
2700 Willow St.
North Little Rock, AR 72115
(501) 758-1516

Veterans Administration Hospital
Drug Dependence Treatment
  Center
North Little Rock, AR 72114
(501) 372-8361

Western Arkansas Counseling
  and Guidance Center
Ozark Clinic
Ozark, AR 72949
(501) 667-2497

Ozark Guidance Center
Springdale Center
Springdale, AR 72764
(501) 751-7052

California
Anaheim Psychological Center
1695 W. Crescent Ave.
Anaheim, CA 92801
(714) 956-2000

Sierra View
366 Elm

Auburn, CA 95603
(916) 885-7561

Kernview Mental Health Center
 and Hospital
3600 San Dimas St.
Bakersfield, CA 93301
(805) 327-7621

Baldwin Park Self-Help Center
4640 Main Ave.
Baldwin Park, CA 91706
(213) 962-6913

Brea Hospital Neuro-Psychiatric
 Center
875 N. Brea Blvd.
Brea, CA 92621
(714) 529-4963

Mercy San Juan Hospital
Care Unit
6501 Coyle Ave.
Carmichael, CA 95608
(916) 961-1400

Vista Hill Hospital
3 N. 2nd Ave.
Chula Vista, CA 92010
(714) 426-3300

Capistrano by the Sea Hospital
33915 Del Obispo Rd.
Dana Point, CA 92629
(714) 496-5702

Drug Treatment Center
Building 305, Rancho Los Amigos
 Hospital
Downey, CA 90242
(213) 922-7425

Catholic Community Service
497 S. 4th St.
El Centro, CA 92243
(714) 353-1020

Martinez Veterans Administration
Outpatient Treatment Center
Emeryville, CA 94608
(415) 228-6800

Griffin Clinic
5363 Balboa Blvd.
Encino, CA 91316
(213) 788-5123

Homboldt County Community
 Mental Health
2200 Harrison Ave.
Eureka, CA 95501
(707) 443-4511

Glendale Guidance Clinic
417 Arden Ave.
Glendale, CA 91203
(213) 244-7257

Hacienda Heights Psychological
 Center
2219 S. Hacienda Blvd.
Hacienda Heights, CA 91745
(213) 330-6823

Hawthorne Community Hospital
 Psychiatric Unit
11711 S. Grevillea Ave.
Hawthorne, CA 90250
(213) 973-1711

Antelope Valley Hospital Medical
 Center
1600 W. Ave. J
Lancaster, CA 93534
(213) 984-4577

Loma Linda University Hospital
Anderson St. and Barton Rd.
Loma Linda, CA 92354
(714) 796-7311

Navy Alcohol Rehabilitation
 Service
Naval Medical Center
Long Beach, CA 90822
(213) 420-5541

Memorial Hospital Medical
 Center
2801 Atlantic Ave.
Box 1428
Long Beach, CA 90801
(213) 595-2236 or 595-2471

UCLA Neuropsychiatric Institute
Inpatient Detoxification
760 Westwood Plaza
Los Angeles, CA 90024
(213) 825-0233

Viewpark Community Hospital
Careunit Program
5035 Coliseum St.
Los Angeles, CA 90016
(213) 295-5314

Alcoholism Council of Greater
Los Angeles
2001 Beverly Blvd.
Los Angeles, CA 90057
(213) 413-4800

Monte Villa Hospital
Hale and Llagas Rd.
Box 947
Morgan Hill, CA 95037
(408) 779-4151 or 226-3020

El Camino Hospital
2500 Grant Rd.
Mountain View, CA 94940
(415) 968-8111

Raleigh Hills Hospital
1501 E. 16th St.
Newport Beach, CA 92663
(714) 645-5707

Catholic Social Center
433 Jefferson St.
Oakland, CA 94607
(415) 834-5656

Gladman Memorial Hospital
2633 E. 27th St.
Oakland, CA 94607
(415) 536-8111, Ext. 240 or 244 or
246

Desert Hospital Mental Health
Center
Box 1647
Palm Springs, CA 92262
(714) 325-9166

Palmdale General Hospital
Mental Health Division
1212 East Avenue South
Palmdale, CA 93550
(805) 273-2211

North County Mental Health
Center
270 Grant, Rm. 150
Palo Alto, CA 94306
(415) 321-2141, Ext. 381

Pasadena Community Counseling
Center
155 N. Madison
Pasadena, CA 91101
(213) 795-7769

Las Encinas Hospital
2900 E. Del Mar Boulevard
Pasadena, CA 91107
(213) 795-9901

St. Luke Hospital Care Unit
2632 E. Washington Blvd.
Pasadena, CA 91107
(213) 797-1141

Behavioral Health Services
1603 Aviation Blvd.
Redondo Beach, CA 90278
(213) 673-5750

Riverside County General
Hospital
Psychiatric Unit
Riverside, CA 92503
(714) 689-2211

Sunny Hills
300 Sunnyhills Dr.
San Anselmo, CA 94960
(415) 457-3200

Center for Dependent Behavior
686 E. Mill St.
San Bernardino, CA 92405
(714) 824-0800

Gifford Mental Health Clinic
3427 4th Ave.

San Diego, CA 92103
(714) 299-3580

Southeast Counseling and
Consultant Service
5835 Imperial Ave.
San Diego, CA 92114
(714) 262-0280

Western Institute of Human
Resources
7522 Clairemont Mesa Blvd.
San Diego, CA 92111
(714) 292-4220

Alcoholism Clinic
Presbyterian Hospital of Pacific
Medical Center
2324 Sacramento St.
San Francisco, CA 94115
(415) 563-4321, Ext. 2361 or 2362

Center for Special Problems
2107 Van Ness Ave.
San Francisco, CA 94109
(415) 558-2001

San Francisco Polydrug Project
527 Irving St.
San Francisco, CA 94122
(415) 566-1700

San Francisco General Hospital
Ward 52 and 72
Department of Public Health
San Francisco, CA 94110
(415) 648-6016

Westside Community Mental
Health Center
2209 Sutter St.
San Francisco, CA 94115
(415) 563-7710

Family Counseling Service of
West San Gabriel Valley
1027 S. Gabriel Blvd.
San Gabriel, CA 91776
(209) 754-3819

Central County Mental Health
Center
3700 Edison St.
San Mateo, CA 94402
(415) 573-2929

Family Service of Marin
1005 A St.
San Rafael, CA 94901
(415) 456-3853

Marin Open House, Inc.
1466 Lincoln Ave.
San Rafael, CA 94901
(415) 457-3755

Family Service of Santa Barbara
800 Santa Barbara St.
Santa Barbara, CA 93101
(805) 965-1001

Santa Cruz Community Counseling Center
271 Water St.
Santa Cruz, CA 95060
(408) 423-2003

Care Unit
South Coast Community Hospital
31872 Coast Highway
South Laguna, CA 92677
(714) 499-1311

Sutter County Hospital
1965 Live Oak Blvd.
Yuba City, CA 95991
(916) 742-9274

Colorado
Maytag Clinic, Inc.
1666 Elmira St., Suite 105
Aurora, CO 80010
(303) 343-1587

Boulder Memorial Hospital
Psychiatric Ward
311 Mapleton Ave.
Boulder, CO 80302
(303) 443-0230

Day At A Time Alcoholism
  Treatment Unit
Boulder Psychiatric Institute
4390 Baseline Rd.
Boulder, CO 80303
(303) 444-2238

Mental Health Center of Boulder
  County
1333 Iris Ave.
Boulder, CO 80302
(303) 443-8500

St. Francis Hospital
800 E. Pike's Peak Ave.
Colorado Springs, CO 80903
(303) 473-6830

Denver Department of Health
  and Hospitals
Mental Health Center
West 8th Ave. and Cherokee St.
Denver, CO 80204
(303) 893-7533 or 893-7566

St. Luke's Hospital
601 E. 19th Ave.
Denver, CO 80203
(303) 292-0600, Ext. 2621

The Harmony Foundation
Box 1989
Estes Park, CO 80517
(303) 586-4491

Connecticut
University of Connecticut
  Health Center
Dempsey Hospital
Alcohol Treatment Program
Farmington, CT 06032
(203) 674-3422

Blue Hills Hospital Inpatient Unit
51 Coventry St.
Hartford, CT 06112
(203) 566-3390

Institute of Living
200 Retreat Ave.
Hartford, CT 06106
(203) 278-7950

High Watch Farm
Carter Rd.
Box 206
Kent, CT 06757
(203) 927-3772

Silver Hill Foundation
Valley Rd.
New Canaan, CT 06840
(203) 966-3561

Fairfield Hills Hospital
Edon House
Newtown, CT 06470
(203) 426-2531

Norwich Hospital Outpatient
  Clinic
110 Broadway
Norwich, CT 06360

Starlite Farm
Box 218
North Stonington, CT 06359
(203) 535-1010

Norwalk Hospital
Alcoholism Rehabilitation
  Program
24 Stevens St.
Norwalk, CT 06850
(203) 838-3611

Delaware
Newark Counseling Center
349 E. Main St.
Newark, DE 19711
(302) 738-7411

Limen House for Women
624 N. Broom St.
Wilmington, DE 19805
(302) 652-9510

The Wilmington Counseling
Center
1327 Washington St.
Wilmington, DE 19801
(302) 571-3500

Wilmington Medical Center
Clinic on Alcoholism
505 W. 13th St.
Wilmington, DE 19801
(302) 428-6276 or 428-6275

District of Columbia

Psychiatric Institution Drug
Center
2101 K St., N.W.
Washington, D.C. 20037
(202) 467-4600

Veterans Administration
Community Clinic
3103 Georgia Ave., N.W.
Washington, D.C. 20010
(202) 483-6666

Florida

Bowling Green Inn, Inc.
U.S. 17 North
Box 337
Bowling Green, FL 33834
(813) 375-2218

Delray Problem Center
170 N.W. 5th Ave.
Delray Beach, FL 33444
(305) 278-0044

Family Study Center
13132 Barwick Rd.
Delray Beach, FL 33444
(305) 278-6275

Coral Ridge Psychiatric Hospital
4545 N. Federal Highway
Fort Lauderdale, FL 33308
(305) 771-2711

General Hospital of Fort Walton
Beach
1000 Marwalt Dr.

Fort Walton Beach, FL 32548
(904) 242-1111

Consultation and Guidance
Service, and Gestalt Institute
of North Florida
412 N.E. 16th Ave., Suite 10
Gainesville, FL 32601
(904) 376-2427

Martin LaZoritz, M.D., Director
Shands Teaching Hospital
University of Florida
Gainesville, FL 32611
(904) 392-3601

Operation Self-Help, Inc.
950 E. 56th St.
Hialeah, FL 33013
(305) 685-0391

Catholic Service Bureau Drug
Program
3211 Flagler Ave.
Key West, FL 33040
(305) 296-8032

In-Patient Detoxification Unit
Jackson Memorial Hospital
Miami, FL 33136
(305) 325-6696

F. L. Dodge Memorial Hospital
1861 N.W. South River Dr.
Miami, FL 33125
(305) 642-3555

Open House Foundation
1566 S.W. First St.
Miami, FL 33135
(305) 643-1593

Bay Memorial Medical Center
600 N. MacArthur Ave.
Panama City, FL 32401
(904) 769-1511

South Miami Hospital
Attn: Dolores A. Morgan, M.D.
7400 S.W. 62nd Ave.
South Miami, FL 33143
(305) 661-4611, Ext. 3871

Family Service Association of
  Greater Tampa
Suite 23, Riverside Professional
  Building
Tampa, FL 33606
(813) 253-0531

Community Mental Health
  Center
Substance Abuse Program
West Palm Beach, FL 33407
(305) 844-9741

Gratitude Guild, Inc.
317 N. Lakeside Court
West Palm Beach, FL 33407
(305) 833-6826 or 833-9232

Georgia
Georgia Mental Health Institute
1256 Briarcliff Rd., N.E.
Atlanta, GA 30306

The Dekalb Addiction Clinic
1260 Briarcliff Rd., N.E.
Atlanta, GA 30306
(404) 894-5771

Peachford Hospital
Alcoholism Program
2151 Peachford Rd.
Atlanta, GA 30338
(404) 455-3200

Georgia Regional Hospital at
  Augusta
3405 Old Savannah Rd.
Augusta, GA 30906
(404) 790-2310

N.W. Georgia Mental Health
  Center
Hutcheson Memorial Tri-County
  Hospital
Fort Oglethorpe, GA 30742
(404) 861-1416

Alcoholism and Drug Unit
Central State Hospital
Milledgeville, GA 31062
(912) 453-5133

Clayton Mental Health Center
15 S.W. Upper Riverdale Rd.
Riverdale, GA 30274
(404) 471-4111

Hawaii
East Hawaii Mental Health
  Services
37 Kekaulike St.
Hilo, HI 96720
(808) 935-3709

Child and Family Service
200 N. Vineyard Blvd.
Honolulu, HI 96817
(808) 521-2377

Koko Head Mental Health Clinic
Honolulu, HI 96816
(808) 735-2448

Maui Memorial Hospital
221 Mahalani St.
Wailuku, HI 96793
(808) 244-9056, Ext. 141 or 160

Kaneohe Mental Health Clinic
Kaneohe, HI 96744
(808) 247-2148

The Habilitat, Inc.
45-035 Kuhonu Pl.
Kaneohe, HI 96744
(808) 235-3691

Idaho
Codac (Community Coordination
  on Drug Abuse Control)
700 Robbins Rd.
Boise, ID 83702
(208) 336-1630

Idaho Regional Treatment and
  Training Center

Box 541
Gooding, ID 83330

Institute of Daily Living
Weiser, ID 83672
(208) 549-2552

Illinois
Mercy Center for Health Care
   Services
1325 N. Highland Ave.
Aurora, IL 60506
(312) 859-2222, Ext. 206

Alternatives Inc.
2546 W. Peterson Ave.
Chicago, IL 60659

City of Chicago Department of
   Health
Civic Center, 2853
Chicago, IL 60602
(312) 744-8174

Chicago Lakeshore Hospital
Alcoholism Treatment Unit
4840 N. Marine Dr.
Chicago, IL 60640

Gateway Houses Foundation, Inc.
505 N. LaSalle St.
Chicago, IL 60610
(312) 822-0032

Lutheran Welfare Services of
   Illinois
4840 W. Byron St.
Chicago, IL 60641
(312) 282-7800

Rush-Presbyterian
St. Luke's Medical Center
Sheridan Rd. Pavilion
6130 N. Sheridan Rd.
Chicago, IL 60660
(312) 743-2171

Metro East Medical and
   Psychiatric Services

333 N. Ninth
East St. Louis, IL 62201
(618) 271-1638

Naval Alcohol Rehabilitation
   Service
Bureau of Naval Personnel (PC6)
Building 200H Ward 7S
Great Lakes, IL
(312) 688-6890

Lutheran General Hospital
1775 Dempster St.
Park Ridge, IL 60068
(312) 696-6050

Loyola University
Foster G. McGaw Hospital
2160 S. First Ave.
Maywood, IL 60153
(312) 531-3750

Comprehensive Mental Health
   Board
Douglas Hall
East Peoria, IL 61611
(309) 694-4394

Oakwood Manor Comprehensive
   Care Center
3301 W. Richwoods Blvd.
Peoria, IL 61604
(309) 685-5241

Psychological Services Region 3
1225 Larchmont
Springhill, IL 62704
(217) 546-7428

The Family Service Center
1167 Wilmette Ave.
Wilmette, IL 60091
(312) 251-7350

Indiana
Human Aid Center
211 E. 10th St.
Anderson, IN 46016
(317) 644-6655

South Central Community
Mental Health Center
640 S. Rogers
Bloomington, IN 47401
(812) 339-1691

S.W. Indiana Mental Health
Center
Clinical/Medical
415 Mulberry St.
Evansville, IN 47713
(812) 423-7791

Samaritan Health Center
200 E. Beardsley Ave.
Elkhart, IN 46514
(219) 262-3597

Lake County Mental Health
Clinic
4801 W. 5th Ave.
Gary, IN 46406
(219) 949-9031

Fairbanks Hospital, Inc.
1575 Northwestern Ave.
Indianapolis, IN 46202
(317) 638-1574

Indiana University Medical
Center
1100 W. Michigan St.
Indianapolis, IN 46202
(317) 264-7422

Koala Center
1711 Lafayette Ave.
Lebanon, IN 46052
(317) 482-3711

Vincennes Comprehensive
Mental Health Center
Good Samaritan Hospital
Vincennes, IN 47591
(812) 885-3291

Iowa
Chemical Dependency Atlantic
Cass County Memorial Hospital
Atlantic, IA 50022
(712) 328-9506

Chemical Dependency Agency
Council Bluffs Unit
532 First Ave.
Council Bluffs, IA 51501
(712) 328-9506

Chemical Dependency Glenwood
112 N. Walnut St.
Glenwood, IA 51534
(712) 382-9506

Alcoholism Coordination Center
101 S. Taylor
Mason City, IA 50401
(712) 225-2594

Northwest Alcoholism and Drug
Treatment
Spirit Lake, IA 51360
(712) 262-5273

Kansas
Alcohol Consultation and
Treatment Services (ACT)
501½ Commercial
Emporia, KS 66801
(316) 342-0548

University of Kansas Medical
Center
39th and Rainbow Blvd.
Kansas City, KS 66103
(913) 831-6493

Wyandott Mental Health
Center Inc.
36th and Eaton
Kansas City, KS 66103
(913) 831-9500

Menninger Foundation
Alcoholism Recovery Program
Box 829
Topeka, KS 66601
(913) 234-9566

Topeka-Shawnee County Health
Department
1615 W. 8th Ave.

Topeka, KS 66606
(913) 233-5141

Valley Hope Association Alcohol
  Counseling
110 E. Waterman St.
Wichita, KS 67202
(913) 927-5111

Kentucky
Lansdowne Mental Health Center
2162 Greenup Avenue
Box 790
Ashland, KY 41101
(606) 324-1141

Benton Mental Health Center
1300 Olive St.
Benton, KY 42025
(502) 527-1434

Cumberland River Comprehensive
  Care Center
Box 568, American Greetings Rd.
Corbin, KY 40701
(606) 528-7010

Bluegrass West Comprehensive
  Care Center
404 Ann St.
Frankfort, KY 40601
(502) 223-2181

Carter County Mental Health
  Center
115 N. Hord St.
Grayson, KY 41143
(606) 474-9229

Shalomwald, Inc.
507 Yager Ave.
La Grange, KY 40031
(502) 222-7148

Newport Comprehensive Care
718 Columbia St.

Newport, KY 41071
(606) 431-3052

Community Mental Health
  Centers of Western Kentucky
1530 Lone Oak Rd.
Paducah, KY 42001
(502) 442-7121

Marantha Christian Center
140 Highland Blvd.
Paducah, KY 42001
(502) 444-6766

Elliot County Mental Health
  Center
Box 215
Sandy Hook, KY 41171
(606) 738-6163

Comprehensive Care Center
124-126 Professional Ave.
Winchester, KY 40391
(606) 744-2562

Louisiana
Baton Rouge
General Chemical Dependency
  Unit
4040 North Blvd.
Baton Rouge, LA 70806
(504) 387-7970

West Jefferson Mental Health
  Center
2108 8th St.
Harvey, LA 70058
(504) 367-0485

St. Patrick's Hospital
524 S. Ryan
Lake Charles, LA 70601
(318) 436-2511

Answer Desk
Rm. 1W06
City Hall
New Orleans, LA 70112
(504) 586-4431

District I Headquarters
Louisiana Bureau of Substance
  Abuse
3934 Canal St.
New Orleans, LA 70119
(504) 568-5531

Sara Mayo Alcoholism Treatment
  Center
625 Jackson Ave.
New Orleans, LA 70130
(504) 581-1811

Pontchartrain Mental Health
  Center
1190 Florida Ave.
New Orleans, LA 70119
(504) 944-6711

Tulane University School of
  Medicine
Department of Psychiatry and
  Neurology
New Orleans, LA 70112
(504) 588-5405

Maine
OADAP
32 Winthrop St.
Augusta, ME 04330
(207) 289-2781

Eastern Maine Medical Center
489 State St.
Bangor, ME 04401
(207) 947-3711

Milestone Foundation
88 Union Ave.
Old Orchard Beach, ME 04064
(207) 934-9615

Maryland
Psychological Services, Inc.
Institute for Treatment of Alcohol
  and Drug Dependency
111 Annapolis St.
Annapolis, MD 21401
(301) 261-1449 or 263-8255

Gundry Hospital
2 N. Wickam Rd.
Baltimore, MD 21229
(301) 644-9917

Lutheran Hospital of Maryland
730 Ashburton St.
Baltimore, MD 21216
(301) 945-1600

Hidden Brook Treatment Center
Thomas Run Rd.
Bel Air, MD 21014
(301) 879-1919

Howard County Health
  Department
8293 Main St.
Ellicott City, MD 21043
(301) 992-2340

Taylor Manor Hospital
College Ave.
Ellicott City, MD 21043
(301) 465-3322

Community Mental Health
500 W. Patrick St.
Frederick, MD 21701
(301) 662-6123

Brook Lane Psychiatric Center
Box 1945
Hagerstown, MD 21740
(301) 733-0330, Ext. 32

Montgomery General Hospital
Upper Montgomery Community
  Mental Health Center
18101 Prince Philip Dr.
Olney, MD 20832
(301) 774-7800, Ext. 206 or 207

Massachusetts
Franklin County Mental Health
  Association
Amity St.
Amherst, MA 01002
(413) 253-2591

Carney Hospital
2100 Dorchester Ave.
Boston, MA 02124
(617) 296-4000

Massachusetts General Hospital
33 Fruit St.
Boston, MA 02114
(617) 726-2906 or 726-2712

New England Medical Center
   Drug Program
260 Tremont St.
Boston, MA 02116
(617) 482-2800

Family Counseling and Guidance
   Center Inc.
40 Independence Ave.
Braintree, MA 02169
(617) 848-7840

Human Resource Institute
227 Babcock St.
Brookline, MA 02146
(617) 734-5930

Cambridge Hospital Department
   of Psychiatry
1493 Cambridge St.
Cambridge, MA 02139
(617) 354-2020

The Sanctuary Inc.
74 Mt. Auburn St.
Cambridge, MA 02138
(617) 661-0600

Franklin County Public Hospital
Beacon St.
Greenfield, MA 01301
(413) 772-6388

Providence Hospital
1233 Main St.
Holyoke, MA 01040
(413) 536-5111

Marblehead Community
   Counseling Center Inc.
66 Clifton St.
Marblehead, MA 01945
(617) 631-8273

Nantucket Cottage Hospital
S. Prospect St.
Nantucket, MA 02554
(617) 228-1200

Berkshire Medical Center
Pittsfield General Unit
379 East St.
Pittsfield, MA 01201
(413) 442-2786

Family Advocacy Project
Life Resource Center
Pittsfield, MA 01209
(413) 443-6473

Mercy Hospital
233 Caren
Springfield, MA 01104
(413) 739-4751

Springfield Hospital Drug
   Counseling Center
759 Chestnut St.
Springfield, MA 01107
(413) 787-4235

Wareham Area Counseling
   Service Inc.
21 Sandwich Rd.
Wareham, MA 02571
(617) 295-3634

Choate Memorial Hospital
21 Warren Ave.
Woburn, MA 01801
(617) 933-6700

Family Service Organization of
   Worcester, Inc.
31 Harvard St.
Worcester, MA 01608
(617) 756-4646

Fairlawn Hospital, Inc.
189 May St.
Worcester, MA 01602
(617) 754-4102

Michigan
Catholic Social Services
117 North Division
Ann Arbor, MI 48108
(313) 662-4534

Child and Family Services
2301 Platt Rd.
Ann Arbor, MI 48104
(313) 971-6520

Allegan County Community
  Mental Health
Substance Abuse Treatment
  Services
Allegan, MI 49010
(616) 673-6617

Brighton Hospital
Alcoholism Treatment Program
12851 E. Grand River
Brighton, MI 48116
(313) 227-1211

Davison Hotline Human Services
  Center
404 Dayton St.
Davison, MI 48423
(313) 653-3555

Ford Motor Company Drug and
  Alcohol Abuse Program
3001 Miller Rd.
Dearborn, MI 48209
(313) 322-3092

Grateful Home, Inc.
335 E. Grand Blvd.
Detroit, MI 48207
(313) 579-0417

Hutzel Hospital Crisis
  Intervention
4827 Brush St.
Detroit, MI 48201
(313) 494-7041

Midwest Mental Health Clinic
6245 Inkster
Garden City, MI 48135
(313) 421-3300

Kent Community Hospital Care
  Unit
750 Fuller Ave., N.E.
Grand Rapids, MI 49503
(616) 774-3349

Our Hope Association
324 Lyon St., N.E.
Grand Rapids, MI 49503
(616) 451-4187

Pine Rest Christian Hospital
6850 South Division Ave.
Grand Rapids, MI 49508
(616) 455-5000

Glass House Rehabilitation
  Program
419 N. Logan
Lansing, MI 48915
(517) 489-2122

Mercy Hospital Substance Abuse
  Unit
1500 E. Sherman Blvd.
Muskegon, MI 49443
(616) 739-9341

Alternative Lifestyles, Inc.
3297 Orchard Lake Rd.
Orchard Lake, MI 48033
(313) 681-7112

St. Joseph Mercy Hospital
900 Woodward Ave.
Pontiac, MI 48053
(313) 858-3000

Northpoint Intervention Center
10514 W. Jefferson
River Rouge, MI 48174
(313) 224-6746

Catholic Family Service
710 N. Michigan Ave.
Saginaw, MI 48602

Heritage Hospital
24755 Haig
Taylor, MI 48180
(313) 295-3524

Minnesota
Hazelden Foundation Inc.
Box 11
Center City, MN 55012
(612) 257-7184

Minneapolis
Center for Behavior Modification, Inc.
3001 University Ave., S.E.
Minneapolis, MN 55414
(612) 331-3998

Chrysalis
2104 Stevens Ave. South
Minneapolis, MN 55404
(612) 817-0118

Hennepin County Alcohol and
Inebriety Program
527 Park Ave. South
Minneapolis, MN 55414
(612) 348-7994

The Johnson Institute
7325 Wayzata Blvd.
Minneapolis, MN 55426
(612) 544-4165

North Memorial Hospital Crisis
Intervention
3220 Lowery Ave. North
Minneapolis, MN 55422
(612) 588-0616

Pine Manors
Route #2
Nevis, MN 56467
(218) 732-4337

Alcoholism and Drug
Dependence Unit
Rochester Methodist Hospital
and Mayo Clinic
Rochester, MN 55901
(507) 282-4461, Ext. 5371

St. Louis Park Treatment Center
3705 Park Center Blvd.
St. Louis Park, MN 55426
(612) 929-5531

St. Paul-Ramsey Hospital and
Medical Center
640 Jackson St.
St. Paul, MN 55101
(612) 221-3928 or 221-3947

Mississippi
Gulf Coast Family Counseling
1145 W. Howard Ave.
Biloxi, MS 39530
(601) 435-4584

Center for Mental Health
Box 1046
Clarksdale, MS 38614
(601) 627-7267

Community Mental Health
1654 E. Union St.
Greenville, MS 38701
(601) 335-7168

Crossroad Services Inc.
777 N. State St.
Jackson, MS 39205
(601) 969-6969

Jackson Mental Health Center
969 Lakeland Dr.
Jackson, MS 39216
(601) 982-8811

Mental Health Complex
North Mississippi Medical Center
Tupelo, MS 38801
(601) 842-3632

Missouri
Mid-Missouri Alcoholism Center
Mid-Missouri Mental Health
Center
Columbia, MO 65201
(314) 449-2511

Alcohol and Drug Treatment
Center
Farmington State Hospital
Farmington, MO 63640
(314) 756-4586

Fulton State Alcoholism Center
Fulton State Hospital
Fulton, MO 65251
(314) 642-3311

Mark Twain Mental Health
Center
109 Virginia St.
Hannibal, MO 63401
(314) 221-2120

Psychiatric In-patient Unit
109 Virginia
Hannibal, MO 63401
(314) 221-2120

Ozark Community Mental
Health Center
2808 Picher Ave.
Joplin, MO 64801
(417) 781-2410

Greater Kansas City Mental
Health Foundation
600 E. 22nd St.
Kansas City, MO 64108
(816) 471-3000

Members Assistance Program
United Labor Committee of
Missouri
2727 Main, Suite 301
Kansas City, MO 64108
(816) 471-8588

Task Force on Women Alcoholics
Center
3718 Tracy
Kansas City, MO 64109
(816) 931-6359

Nevada State Hospital Alcohol
and Drug Abuse Program
Drawer 308

Nevada, MO 64772
(417) 667-7833

Family Guidance Center
Alcohol and Drug Program
923 Powell St.
St. Joseph's Hospital
St. Joseph, MO 64501
(816) 364-1501

Christian Hospital Northwest
Alcohol Rehabilitation Center
1225 Graham Rd.
St. Louis, MO 63031
(314) 839-3800, Ext. 394

Edgewood Hospital
4201 McKibbon Rd.
St. Louis, MO 63134
(314) 427-1650

Lindell Hospital
4930 Lindell Blvd.
St. Louis, MO 63108
(314) 367-3770, Ext. 220 or 218

Lutheran Medical Center
Chemical Dependency Unit
2939 Miami St.
St. Louis, MO 63118
(314) 772-1456

Personalized Alcoholism
Treatment
Compton Hill Medical Center
1775 S. Grand Blvd.
St. Louis, MO 63104
(314) 771-0500

Montana

Open Door
122 E. Park Ave.
Anaconda, MT 59711
(406) 563-5248

South Central Montana Regional
Mental Health Center
1245 N. 29th
Billings, MT 59101
(406) 252-3851

Gallatin Council on Health and
  Drugs
15 S. Tract St.
Bozeman, MT 59715
(440) 672-3651

Southwest Montana Mental
  Health Center
225 S. Idaho
Butte, MT 59701
(406) 723-3447

Hilltop Recovery, Inc.
1020 Assiniboine Ave.
Havre, MT 59501
(406) 265-9665

Eastern Montana Regional
  Mental Health Center
Executive Building
Miles City, MT 59301
(406) 232-1687

Nebraska

Mid Nebraska Mental Health
  Center
914 Bauman
Grand Island, NE 68801
(402) 471-2691

Lincoln Council on Alcoholism
  and Drugs
215 S. 15th St.
Lincoln, NE 68508
(402) 475-2694

Nebraska Methodist Hospital
Chemical Dependency Unit
36th and Cuming Streets
Omaha, NE 68131
(402) 397-3150, Ext. 521

Nebraska Psychiatric Institute
602 S. 45th St.
Omaha, NE 68106
(402) 541-4870

Pioneer Mental Health Center
729 Seward St.

Seward, NE 68434
(402) 643-3343

Nevada

Las Vegas Mental Health Center
6161 W. Charlestown
Las Vegas, NV 89102
(702) 870-7211

North Las Vegas Hospital
Careunit Program
1409 E. Lake Mead Blvd.
North Las Vegas, NV 89030
(702) 642-6905

Sunrise Hospital
Medical Center
3186 Maryland Parkway
Box 14157
Las Vegas, NV 89114
(702) 731-8000

Alcoholics Rehabilitation
  Association
2550 Dickerson Rd.
Reno, NV 89503
(702) 786-9917

Nevada Mental Health Institute
Box 2460
Reno, NV 89505
(702) 322-6961, Ext. 351 or 350

New Hampshire

The Counseling Center of
  Sullivan County
Box 1219
18 Bailey Ave.
Claremont, NH 03743
(603) 542-2578

New Hampshire Hospital
105 Pleasant St.
Concord, NH 03301
(603) 224-6531

Beech Hill Farm
Box 234
Dublin, NH 03444
(603) 563-8511

Dartmouth-Hitchcock Mental
Health Center
9 Maynard St.
Hanover, NH 03755
(603) 643-4000, Ext. 3667

North Conway Memorial
Hospital
Alcohol and Drug Abuse Program
North Conway, NH 03860
(603) 356-5461 or 569-1884

New Jersey
Integrity House
John E. Runnels Hospital
Berkley Heights, NJ 07922
(201) 322-7240

Together, Inc.
7 State St.
Glassboro, NJ 08028
(609) 881-4040

Mountainside Hospital
Bay and Highland Avenues
Montclair, NJ 07042
(201) 746-6000, Ext. 360 or 252

Morristown Memorial Hospital
100 Madison Ave.
Morristown, NJ
(201) 540-5238

Burlington County Memorial
Hospital
175 Madison Ave.
Mt. Holly, NJ 08060

Martland Alcoholism Treatment
Center
116 Fairmount Ave.
Newark, NJ 07107

New Jersey College of Medicine
Drug Treatment Center
15 Roseville Ave.
Newark, NJ 07107
(201) 482-8702, Ext. 54

Family Service and Child Guidance Center
395 S. Center St.
Orange, NJ 07050
(201) 675-3817

Bergen Pines County Hospital
E. Ridgewood Ave.
Paramus, NJ 07652
(201) 261-9000, Ext. 593

Seabrook House
Box 55
705 Polk Lane
Seabrook, NJ 08302
(609) 455-7575

Hill House
Overlook Hospital
193 Morris Ave.
Summit, NJ 07901
(201) 522-2000

Fair Oaks Hospital
19 Prospect St.
Summit, NJ 07901
(201) 277-0143

New Mexico
Bernalillo County Mental Health
Center
2600 Marble N.E.
Albuquerque, NM 87106
(505) 265-3511

Vista Sandia Hospital
501 Richfield Ave. N.E.
Albuquerque, NM 87113
(505) 898-1661

Community Mental Health
Services
414 W. Mermod St.
Carlsbad, NM 88220
(505) 887-1324

Mental Health Resources Inc.
815 West 2nd
Clovis, NM 88101
(505) 762-6394

Southwest Mental Health Center
575 N. Main St.
Las Cruces, NM 88001
(505) 526-6604

Los Alamos Family Council
Los Alamos, NM 87544
(505) 662-3264

Greater Santa Rose Council on
    Alcoholism
437 S. 4th St.
Santa Rosa, NM 88435
(505) 472-5383

Grant County ACERT Program
Box 677
Silver City, NM 88061
(505) 388-4412

New York
Drug Dependence Treatment
    Center Administration
VA Hospital
113 Holland Ave.
Albany, NY 12208
(518) 462-3311

SUNY Middle Earth
400 Washington Ave.
Albany, NY 12203
(518) 457-7588

Brunswick Hospital Center
366 Broadway
Amityville, NY 11701
(516) 264-5000, Ext. 361

South Oaks Hospital
Box 426
Amityville, NY 11701
(516) 264-4000, Ext. 319

Craig House Hospital
Howland Ave.

Beacon, NY 12508
(914) 831-1200

Bronx-Lebanon Hospital Center
321 E. Tremont Ave.
Bronx, NY 10457
(212) 583-6363

Hunts Point Multi-Service Center
630 Jackson Ave.
Bronx, NY 10455
(212) 993-3000, Ext. 279 or 252

Riverdale Mental Health Clinic
2736 Independence Ave.
Bronx, NY 10463
(212) 796-5300

Brooklyn Hospital Medical
    Center
121 Dekalb Ave.
Brooklyn, NY 11201
(212) 270-4411

Coney Island Hospital
2601 Ocean Parkway
Brooklyn, NY 11235
(212) 934-9800

Kings County Hospital —
    K Building
600 Albany Ave.
Brooklyn, NY 11203
(212) 630-4520 or 630-4507

Buffalo Psychiatric Center
400 Forest Ave.
Buffalo, NY 14213
(716) 885-2261

Bry-Lin Hospital
1263 Delaware Ave.
Buffalo, NY 14209
(716) 886-8200, Ext. 153

YMCA South Buffalo Counseling
    Center
457 Abbott Rd.
Buffalo, NY 14220
(716) 824-0867

Stepping Stones Farm
Peekskill Hollow Rd.
Carmel, NY 10512
(914) 225-3109

Clifton Springs Hospital and
Clinic
2 Coulter Rd.
Clifton Springs, NY 14432
(315) 462-9561

Mount Sinai Hospital Services
Alcoholism Treatment Program
City Hospital at Elmhurst
79-01 Broadway
Elmhurst, NY 11373
(212) 830-1371

Long Island Jewish Medical
Center
327 Beach 19th St.
Far Rockaway, NY 11691
(516) 471-8100

Family Community Center
17 Buffalo Ave.
Freeport, NY 11520
(516) 378-8666

Warren Washington Community
Mental Health Center
Glen Falls Hospital
Glen Falls, NY 12801
(518) 793-5148

Strauss Cottage
Long Island Jewish Hillside
Medical Center
Glen Oaks, NY 11004
(212) 343-6700

Family Service Association
129 Jackson St.
Hempstead, NY 11550
(516) 485-4600

Jewish Community Services of
Long Island
50 Clinton St.
Hempstead, NY 11550
(516) 485-5710

Queens Hospital Center
82-68 164th St.
Jamaica, NY 11432

Samuel Field YM-YWHA
58-20 Little Neck Parkway
Little Neck, NY 11362
(212) 225-6750

Casa Serena
Watermelon Hill Rd.
Mahopac, NY 10541
(914) 628-9622 or 628-9823

North Nassau Mental Health
Center
1691 Northern Blvd.
Manhasset, NY 11030
(516) 627-7550 or 627-7530

North Shore University Hospital
300 Community Dr.
Manhasset, NY 11030
(516) 562-4665

Bernstein Institute
341 E. 25th St.
New York, NY 10010
(212) 689-6709

Gracie Square Hospital
420 E. 76th St.
New York, NY 10021
(212) 988-4400

Greenwich House Counseling
Center
116 W. 14th St.
New York, NY 10011
(212) 691-2900

International Center Integrative
Studies
The Door
New York, NY 10011
(212) 691-2960

New York Medical College
Department of Psychiatry
New York, NY 10029
(212) 369-7900

Psychobiology Study Unit
Payne Whitney Clinic, New York
  Hospital
525 E. 68th St.
New York, NY 10021
(212) 472-6430

Rockefeller University
York Ave. and 66th St.
New York, NY 10012
(212) 360-1000

Roosevelt Hospital Smithers
  Alcoholism Facility
56 E. 93rd St.
New York, NY 10028
(212) 369-9566

Roosevelt Hospital Substance
  Abuse Program
428 W. 59th St.
Manhattan, NY 10019
(212) 554-6570

St. Vincent's Hospital —
  Manhattan
201 W. 13th St.
New York, NY 10011
(212) 924-0756 or 620-2061

Niagara County Mental Health
  Services
910 Ferry Ave.
Niagara Falls, NY 14301
(716) 285-9636

Oceanside Counseling Center
Foxhurst Rd.
Oceanside, NY 11572
(516) 766-6283

Youth and Family Counseling
  Agency
193 South St.
Oyster Bay, NY 11771
(516) 922-6867

The Rhinebeck Lodge for
  Successful Living

RD 1, Milan Hollow Rd.
Rhinebeck, NY 12572
(914) 266-5777

United Hospital
Boston Post Rd.
Port Chester, NY 10573
(914) 939-7000, Ext. 204

University of Rochester —
  Medical Center
300 Crittenden Blvd.
Rochester, NY 14642
(716) 275-3535

Rochester Mental Health Center
1425 Portland Ave.
Rochester, NY 14621
(716) 544-5220

Rochester Psychiatric Center
1600 South Ave.
Rochester, NY 14620

St. Vincent's Hospital — Staten
  Island
111 Water St.
Staten Island, NY 10304
(212) 448-3978

SE Nassau Guidance Center
3375 Park Ave.
Wantagh, NY 11793
(516) 781-1911

Sleepy Valley Farms
Warwick, NY 10990
(914) 986-2545 or 986-9506

The Family Switchboard
16 Rock City Rd.
Woodstock, NY 12498

North Carolina
Stanly Center
Box 1396
Albermarle, NC 28001
(704) 983-2117

Alcohol Rehabilitation Program
Western Carolina Hospital
Box 1058
Black Mountain, NC 28711
(704) 669-6411, Ext. 400

Department of Psychiatry
505 N. Church St.
Chapel Hill, NC 27514
(919) 966-4285

Charlotte Treatment Center
Box 15197
1715 Sharon Rd. West
Charlotte, NC 28210
(704) 544-8373

Cherry Hospital
Highway 581 West
Caller Box 8000
Goldsboro, NC 27530
(919) 731-3451

Mental Health Center
301 N. Herman Street
Box DD
Goldsboro, NC 27530
(919) 736-9110

Department of Psychiatry
Bowman-Gray School of Medicine
North Carolina Baptist Hospital
Winston-Salem, NC 27103
(919) 727-4552

Mandala Center
Reynolds Memorial Hospital
Winston-Salem, NC 27101
(919) 724-9236

Alcoholism Resident Care
    Authority
Box 12308
Union Cross Rd.
Winston-Salem, NC 27101
(919) 784-9470

North Dakota
St. Joseph's Hospital
Alcohol and Drug Abuse
    Treatment Unit

Dickinson, ND 58601
(701) 225-6771, Ext. 229

Alcohol and Drug Dependency
    Unit
St. John's Hospital
Fargo, ND 58102
(701) 232-3331

United Hospital Chemical
    Dependency Unit
1200 S. Columbia Rd. — North
    Unit
Grand Forks, ND 58201
(701) 775-5521

North Dakota State Hospital
Chemical Dependency Unit
Jamestown, ND 58401
(701) 253-2750

St. Joseph's Hospital
SE 3rd and 4th St.
Minot, ND 58701
(701) 838-0341, Ext. 202 or 294

Ohio
Family Values Project
YMCA
80 W. Center St.
Akron, OH 44308

Bay View Hospital
Serenity Hall
23200 Lake Rd.
Bay Village, OH 44140
(216) 331-2500

Health Center
425 Chestnut St.
Chillicothe, OH 45601
(614) 775-1799

Eden House
206 E. William Howard Taft Rd.
Cincinnati, OH 45219
(513) 751-3364

Family Counseling Services
2343 Auburn Ave.

Cincinnati, OH 45219
(513) 381-6300

Cleveland Psychiatric Institute
1708 Aiken Ave.
Cleveland, OH 44109
(216) 661-6200

Riverside Methodist Hospital
3535 Olentangy River Rd.
Columbus, OH 43214
(614) 261-5591

Lorain Community Hospital
3700 Kolbe Rd.
Lorain, OH 44089

Union County Counseling
　Services
Memorial Hospital
Marysville, OH 43040
(513) 644-6115

Alcoholism Program
Lake County General Health
　District
30 Liberty St.
Suite #2
Painesville, OH 44077
(216) 352-6281, Ext. 264 or 273

Portage County Alcoholism
　Services
231 S. Chestnut St.
Ravenna, OH 44266
(216) 297-5829

Shelby County Mental Health
　Clinic
500 E. Court St.
Sidney, OH 45365
(513) 492-4178

Sandusky Valley Mental Health
　Center
67 St. Francis Ave.
Tiffin, OH 44883
(419) 447-8331

Serenity House
Caller No. 10002
Toledo, OH 43699
(419) 381-8355

Toledo Health Dept.
635 N. Erie St.
Toledo, OH 43624
(419) 247-6199

Human Services Center of Wayne
　County
450 N. Market St.
Wooster, OH 44691
(216) 264-9597

Oklahoma
Regional Guidance Center
1630 E. Beverly
Ada, OK 74820
(405) 332-0085

Guidance Clinic of Southern
　Oklahoma
14 K St., S.W.
Ardmore, OK 73401
(405) 223-5636

Bethany Guidance Center
1728 N. Rockwell
Bethany, OK 73008
(405) 789-4801

Durant Community Mental
　Health Clinic
504 Evergreen St.
Durant, OK 74701
(405) 924-4045

Helen Holiday Home, Inc .
411 Gore Blvd.
Lawton, OK 73501
(405) 357-8114

Mid-Del Youth and Family Center
300 Mid-America Blvd.
Midwest City, OK 73110
(405) 737-6668

Muskogee County Guidance
Center
530 S. 34th St.
Muskogee, OK 74401
(918) 687-4456

Central State Griffin Memorial
Hospital
Box 151
Norman, OK 73069
(405) 321-4880, Ext. 524

Norman Community Guidance
Center
909 E. Almameda
Norman, OK 73069
(405) 321-4048

Healthline Information and
Referral
Oklahoma State Department of
Health
N.E. 10th and Stonewall
Box 53551
Oklahoma City, OK 73152
(405) 271-4725

The Harbingers, Inc.
1401 N.E. 70th St.
Oklahoma City, OK 73111
(405) 478-2809

Coyne Campbell Hospital
2601 N. Spencer Rd.
Spencer, OK 73084
(405) 427-2441

Stigler Mental Health Clinic
Box 296
Stigler, OK 74462
(918) 967-8491

Katharyn Cornell School of
Alcohol and Other Drug
Studies
The University of Tulsa
600 S. College
Tulsa, OK 74104

St. John Medical Center Inc.
Alcohol Treatment Center
1923 S. Utica
Tulsa, OK 74104
(918) 744-2502

The Haven
1647 S. Elwood
Tulsa, OK 74119
(918) 585-1389

Southwest Guidance Center
7012 S. Kleiner
Wheatland, OK 73097
(405) 745-3419

Oregon
Buckley House, Inc.
332 W. 5th
Eugene, OR 97401

Serenity Lane, Inc.
Alcoholism Treatment Center
616 E. 16th Ave.
Eugene, OR 97401
(503) 687-1110

Gresham Community Hospital
Careunit Program
N.E. 5th and Beech Streets
Gresham, OR 97030
(503) 667-1122

Interfaith Counseling Center
833 S.W. 11th, Suite 406
Portland, OR 97205
(503) 223-6698

Physicians and Surgeons Hospital
Alcohol Care Unit
1927 N.W. Lovejoy
Portland, OR 97209
(503) 224-6500 or 224-6510

Woodland Park Mental Health
Center
1400 S.E. Umatilla
Portland, OR 97202
(503) 234-5353

Pennsylvania
Gateway Rehabilitation Center
Moffett Run Rd.
Aliquippa, PA 15001
(412) 378-4461

Altoona Hospital Community
    Mental Health Center
700 Howard Ave. and 7th St.
Altoona, PA 16601
(814) 946-2279

The Counseling Service Inc.
441 N. Spring St.
Bellefonte, PA 16823
(814) 355-5541

Family Counseling Service
603 W. Main St.
Bloomsburg, PA 17815
(717) 784-5773

Addictive Behavior Unit
Irene Stacy Mental Health Clinic
112 Hillvue
Butler, PA 16001
(412) 287-0791

Today, Inc.
31 W. Ashland Ave.
Doylestown, PA 18901
(215) 345-6074

Drug and Alcohol Abuse Program
    Community Education Center
133 Hedley Ave.
Dushore, PA 18614
(717) 787-9764

Eagleville Hospital and Rehabili-
    tation
Box 45
Eagleville, PA 19406
(215) 539-6000

Abraxas Foundation Inc.
348 S.W. 8th St.
Erie, PA 16502
(814) 459-0618

St. Vincent Hospital Community
    Health
232 W. 25th St.
Erie, PA 16502
(814) 459-4000

Changing Times Center
2227 Darby Rd.
Havertown, PA 19083
(215) 853-2660

Conemaugh Valley Memorial
    Hospital
1086 Franklin St.
Johnstown, PA 15905
(814) 536-6671

Armstrong County Council on
    Alcohol Problems
301 Arthur St.
Kittanning, PA 16201
(412) 548-7607

Family Counseling Center
Lancaster General Hospital
Lancaster, PA 17604
(717) 299-5511

St. Joseph Hospital
250 College Ave.
Lancaster, PA 17604
(717) 299-5511

Newtown Facility — Today Inc.
Woodbourne Rd.
Langhorne, PA 19047
(215) 968-4713

Abraxas I
The Abraxas Foundation
Box 59
Marienville, PA 16239
(814) 927-6615

Spencer Hospital
1034 Grove St.
Meadville, PA 16335
(814) 337-1261

Today (Newtown Facility)
Box 98
Newtown, PA 18940
(215) 968-4713

Eagleville Halfway House
901 Dekalb St.
Norristown, PA 19406
(215) 279-6100

Paoli Hospital
Lancaster Pike
Paoli, PA 19301
(215) 647-2200

CODAAP
1405 Locust St., 2nd Floor
Philadelphia, PA 19102
(215) 735-0664

Larchwood Counseling Center
5323 Larchwood Ave.
Philadelphia, PA 19143
(215) 747-7373

Philadelphia Psychiatric Center
Ford Rd. and Monument Ave.
Philadelphia, PA 19131
(215) 877-2000

West Philadelphia Community
   Mental Health Consortium Inc.
Cobbs Creek Counseling Center
5923 Walnut St.
Box 8076
Philadelphia, PA 19101
(215) 474-3475

Special Treatment Unit
St. John's General Hospital
Pittsburgh, PA 15212
(412) 766-8300

Families Together
4527 Winthrop St.
Pittsburgh, PA 15213
(412) 621-7877

St. Francis Hospital Community
   Mental Health Center Drug
   Service
45th Off Pennsylvania Ave.
Pittsburgh, PA 15201
(412) 622-4545

Good Samaritan Hospital Alcoholism and Drug Counseling
727 E. Norwegian St.
Pottsville, PA 17901
(717) 622-5898

Alcoholism Treatment Center
12th and Walnut St.
Reading, PA 19103
(215) 376-4901

Chit-Chat Farms
Box 277
Wernersville, PA 19565
(215) 678-2332

Colonial Halfway House
3800 W. Market St.
York, PA 17405
(717) 792-9702

Puerto Rico
Centro de Arecibo
Ave Victor Rojas
Arecibo, PR 00612
(809) 878-4256

Hogar Crea-Barranquitas
Antiguo Hospital Municipal
Barranquitas, PR 00618
(809) 761-0715

Hogar Crea-Mujeres
Carretera a Comerio
Bayamon, PR 00619
(809) 785-8314

Instituto Psicologico de Puerto
   Rico
15 B Avenida Milagros Cabeza
Carolina Alta, PR 00630
(809) 768-3770

Centro Psico-Social Diurno
   Ambulatorio

Calle Zalduondo Veve
Fajardo, PR 00648
(809) 863-3323

Centro de Manati
Road 2 KM 47.7
Manati, PR 00701
(809) 765-5130

Pabellon J y H
Hospital de Psiquiatria Centro
  Medico
Rio Piedras, PR 00928
(809) 765-0575

Casa la Providencia
Boulevard Del Valle 200
Old San Juan, PR 00902
(809) 725-5130

Rhode Island

Washington County Community
  Mental Health Clinic
Old Post Rd.
Box 363
Charlestown, RI 02813
(401) 364-6400

Caritas House
Cottage 404, Cottage Ct A
Cranston, RI 02920
(401) 464-3197

Butler Hospital
345 Blackstone Blvd.
Providence, RI 02906
(401) 456-3700

Providence Mental Health Center
355 Broad St.
Providence, RI 02907
(401) 274-2500

Alcoholism and Family
  Counseling
Warwick Community Action
  Program, Inc.
Box 597
Warwick, RI 02887
(401) 738-1760

South Carolina

Aiken-Barnwell Mental Health
  Center
104 Florence Street S.W.
Aiken, SC 29801
(803) 648-0481

Anderson County Alcohol and
  Drug Abuse Commission
128 W. Benson St.
Anderson, SC 29621
(803) 225-1468

Counseling and Assistance Center
Naval Station
Charleston, SC 29408
(803) 743-5108

Columbia Area Mental Health
  Center
1618 Sunset Dr.
Columbia, SC 29203
(803) 758-2036

South Carolina Alcohol and Drug
  Addiction Center
State Department of Mental
  Health
Columbia, SC 29203
(803) 758-4437

Florence County Commission on
  Alcohol and Drug Abuse
604 Gregg Ave.
Florence, SC 29501
(803) 665-9349

Office of Social Actions
Myrtle Beach Air Force Base, SC
  29577
(803) 238-7069

York County Council on Alcohol/
  Drug Abuse
325 E. White St.
Rock Hill, SC 29730
(803) 327-3118

Union County Commission on
Alcohol and Drug Abuse
Box 844
Union, SC 29379
(803) 427-1241 or 427-1242

South Dakota
Northeastern Mental Health
Center
350 S. State St.
Aberdeen, SD 57401
(605) 225-1010

River Park Center
801 E. Dakota Ave.
Pierre, SD 57501
(605) 224-7331 or 224-5941, Ext.
243

West River Mental Health Center
710 St. Anne St.
Rapid City, SD 57701
(605) 343-7262

Lewis and Clark Mental Health
Center
401 Capitol St.
Yankton, SD 57078
(605) 665-4604

Tennessee
Western Mental Health Institute
Alcohol and Drug Unit
Bolivar, TN 38074
(901) 658-5141, Ext. 279

Bristol Regional Mental Health
Center
26 Midway St.
Bistol, TN 37620
(615) 968-1561

Mocassin Bend Psychiatric
Hospital
Mocassin Bend Rd.
Chattanooga, TN 37405
(615) 265-2271

Harriett Cohn Mental Health
Center

1300 Madison St.
Clarksville, TN 37040
(615) 648-8126

Hiwassee Mental Health Center
755 Broad St.
Cleveland, TN 37116
(615) 479-5454

Covington Mental Health Center
Box 114
Covington, TN 38019
(901) 476-8967

Jackson Council on Alcohol and
Drug Dependency
118 E. Baltimore
Jackson, TN 38301
(901) 423-3653

St. Mary's Medical Center
Oak Hill Ave.
Knoxville, TN 37917
(615) 971-6507

Peninsula Psychiatric Center
Jones Bend Rd.
Maryville, TN 37737
(615) 983-8216

Alcohol and Drug Dependence
Clinic
865 Poplar Ave.
Box 4966
Memphis, TN 38104
(901) 529-7676

Information and Referral Service
3485 Poplar, Suite 1
Memphis, TN 38111
(901) 323-8381

Cumberland Heights
Route 2, River Rd.
Nashville, TN 37209
(615) 352-1/57

Vanderbilt Drug Information-
Treatment-Rehabilitation
Clinic
Vanderbilt University Medical
Center South

Nashville, TN 37212
(615) 322-6605

Regional Mental Health Center
of Oak Ridge
240 W. Tyrone Rd.
Oak Ridge, TN 37830
(615) 482-1076

Multi-County Comprehensive
Mental Health Center
1803 N. Jackson St.
Tullahoma, TN 37388
(615) 455-3476

Texas
The Haven
Amarilla Alcoholic Women's Recovery Center, Inc.
1308 S. Burhanan
Amarillo, TX 79102
(806) 374-9202

Austin Council on Alcoholism
314 W. 11th, Suite 530
Austin, TX 78701
(512) 472-2461

Human Development Center
1430 Collier St.
Austin, TX 78704
(512) 447-4141

Nueces County MH/MR
Substance Abuse Center
615 Oliver Courts
Corpus Christi, TX 78408
(512) 883-1534

Casa Blanca Hospital, Inc.
2345 Reagan St.
Dallas, TX 75219
(214) 521-7541

East Dallas Hospital Program for
Alcoholism, Addictions, Stress,
and Anxiety
6003 Victor
Dallas, TX 75214
(214) 824-7487

Oaklawn Treatment Center
3851 Cedar Springs Rd.
Dallas, TX 75219
(214) 521-6030

R. E. Thomason General Hospital
Box 20009
El Paso, TX 79998
(915) 544-1200, Ext. 285

Family and Individual Services
Association
212 Burnet St.
Fort Worth, TX 76102
(817) 335-2401

Baylor College of Medicine
Alcoholism Treatment Program
Texas Medical Center — Department of Psychiatry
1200 Moursund
Houston, TX 77030
(713) 790-4892

Paasa Houston International
Hospital
6441 Main St.
Houston, TX 77030
(713) 790-0830

Saint Joseph Hospital
Cullen Family Building
1919 Labranch St.
Houston, TX 77002
(713) 225-3131, Ext. 243 or
757-7507

Midland Council on Alcoholism
3701 N. Big Springs
Midland, TX 79701
(915) 682-4721

Mental Health Center for Greater
West Texas
244 N. Magdalin
San Angelo, TX 76901
(915) 655-5676

Villa Rosa Annex
Santa Rosa Medical Center
5115 Medical Dr.
San Antonio, TX 78229

Patrician Movement
222 E. Mitchell
San Antonio, TX 78210
(512) 532-3126

Heart of Texas Mental Health
  Center
1401 North 18
Waco, TX 76703
(817) 752-3451

Utah
Emery County Mental Health
  Center
Professional Building
Castedale, UT 84513
(801) 748-5216

Southern Utah Guidance Center
1552 West 200 North
Cedar City, UT 84720
(801) 586-6341

Family Life Services
Box 309
Cedar City, UT 84720
(801) 586-6341

Northern Utah Mental Health
  Clinic
160 N. Main St.
Logan, UT 84321
(801) 752-3730

Alcohol and Chemical Treatment
  Center
300 Polk Ave.
Ogden, UT 84403
(801) 399-4111

Weber County Mental Health
  Center
350 Healy Ave.
Ogden, UT 84401
(801) 399-8391

Utah Valley Hospital
1034 N. Fifth West
Provo, UT 84601
(801) 373-7850, Ext. 745

Utah State Hospital
Box 270
Provo, UT 84601
(801) 373-4400

Drug Dependence Treatment
  Center, Inpatient
VA Hospital
Salt Lake City, UT 84113
(801) 322-1565

Holy Cross Hospital Psychiatric
  Unit
1045 E. First South
Salt Lake City, UT 84102
(801) 328-9171

LDS Social Services
19 W. South Temple
Salt Lake City, UT 84101
(801) 532-6141

Salt Lake Community Mental
  Health Center
807 E. South Temple
Salt Lake City, UT 84102
(801) 328-0361

University Center
Alcoholism and Drug Abuse
  Clinic
50 N. Medical Dr.
Salt Lake City, UT 84132
(801) 581-6228

The Haven
974 E. South Temple
Salt Lake City, UT 84192
(801) 533-0070

Vermont
Brattleboro Retreat
75 Linden St.
Brattleboro, VT 05301
(802) 254-2331

Alcoholism Information and
Referral
200 North St.
Burlington, VT 05401
(802) 862-5243

Drug Abuse Treatment and
Prevention
Vermont State Hospital
Waterbury, VT 05676
(802) 244-7331

Virgin Islands
St. Croix Rehabilitation Program
153 Richmond
Christiansted, VI 00820
(809) 774-5150

Virginia
Division of Substance Abuse
Alexandria Health Department
515 Wythe St., Rm. 200
Alexandria, VA 22314
(703) 683-6677

Alexandria Mental Health
Association
101 N. Columbus St., Rm. 202
Alexandria, VA 22314
(703) 548-0010

Arlington Hospital
1701 N. George Mason Dr.
Arlington, VA 22205
(703) 558-6536

Prelude
(Alcohol and Drugs)
Main Office, Special Programs
Center
3017 S. 16th St.
Arlington, VA 22204
(703) 920-3410

The David C. Wilson
Neuropsychiatric Hospital
2101 Arlington Blvd.
Charlottesville, VA 22903
(804) 977-1120

Woodburn Center for
Community Mental Health
3340 Woodburn Rd.
Fairfax, VA 22030
(703) 573-0523

Lynchburg Division of
Alcoholism Services
Community Alcohol Services
and Education
405 Bay St.
Lynchburg, VA 24501
(804) 845-7033

Alcohol and Drug Prevention
and Control
Fort Eustis
Newport News, VA 23604
(804) 878-2985

Riverside Hospital
Community Mental Health
Center
Alcoholism Treatment Program
J. Clyde Morris Blvd.
Newport News, VA 23601
(804) 599-2620

Human Resources Institute
100 Kingsley Lane
Norfolk, VA 23505
(804) 489-1072

New River Valley Alcoholism
Recovery Center
Box 3506
Radford, VA 24141
(703) 639-3591

St. Albans Psychiatric Hospital
Box 3608
Radford, VA 24141
(703) 639-2481

Alcohol and Drug Abuse Prevention and Training Services, Inc.
932 W. Franklin St.
Richmond, VA 23220
(804) 358-0408

Richmond VA Hospital
Drug Dependence Treatment
   Center and House of Janus
Richmond, VA 23249
(804) 233-9631

Richmond Division of
   Alcoholism Services
808 W. Main St.
Richmond, VA 23220
(804) 649-8465

Bethany Hall
1109 Franklin Rd., S.W.
Roanoke, VA 24016
(703) 343-4261

White Cross Hospital
Mt. Regis Hill
Salem, VA 24153
(703) 389-4761

Northwestern Community
   Mental Health Center
20 E. Piccadilly St.
Winchester, VA 22601
(703) 667-2488

Washington
Valley Cities Mental Health
   Center
2704 I Street N.E.
Auburn, WA 98002
(206) 854-0760

Eastside Community Mental
   Health Center
2253 140th Ave. N.E.
Bellevue, WA 98005
(206) 747-9000

Dayton General Hospital
1012 S. 3rd St.
Dayton, WA 99328
(509) 382-2531

Evergreen Manor
2605 Summit Ave.
Everett, WA 98201

Alcenas Hospital
10322 N.E. 132nd
Kirkland, WA 98033
(206) 821-1122

Olalla Guest Lodge, Inc.
Route 1, Box 253-C
Olalla, WA 98359
(206) 857-6201

Community Mental Health
2604 12th Court S.W.
Olympia, WA 98502
(206) 943-4760

Memorial Hospital, Inc.
Washington Ave.
Pullman, WA 99163
(509) 332-2541

Care Unit (Comprehensive Care)
Riverton General Hospital
12844 Military Rd., South
Seattle, WA 98168
(206) 244-0180

Harbor View Community Mental
   Health Center
326 9th Ave.
Seattle, WA 98104
(206) 223-3000 or 223-3107

St. Francis Xavier Cabrini
   Hospital
Terry Ave. and Madison St.
Seattle, WA 98104
(206) 623-4254

Studio Club
9010 13th Ave., N.W.
Seattle, WA 98107
(206) 782-2030

Community Personal Guidance
   Center
W. 2308 Third
Spokane, WA 99204
(509) 747-1005

Drug Dependence Treatment
Center
American Lake VA Hospital
Tacoma, WA 98493
(206) 588-2185

Puget Sound Alcoholism Center
Puget Sound Hospital
S. 36th and Pacific Ave.
Tacoma, WA 98408
(206) 474-0533

West Virginia

AR-CAP Program
Beckley Application Reg. Hospital
306 Stanaford Rd.
Beckley, WV 25801
(304) 255-3442

Center on Alcoholism and Drug
Abuse
Number 6 Hospital Plaza
Clarksburg, WV 26301
(304) 623-2986

Center on Alcoholism and Drug
Abuse
300 2nd St.
Box 69
Fairmount, WV 26554
(304) 366-7878

Community Mental Health
Center
3375 U.S. Route 60 East
Huntington, WV 25705
(304) 525-7851

Center on Alcoholism and Drug
Abuse
101 Church St.
Lewisburg, WV 24901
(304) 647-4006

Center on Alcoholism and Drug
Abuse
101 S. Queen St.

Martinsburg, WV 25401
(304) 267-7571

Center on Alcoholism and Drug
Abuse
414 High St.
Morgantown, WV 26505
(304) 296-1731

Center on Alcoholism and Drug
Abuse
1100 Market St.
Parkersburg, WV 26101
(304) 428-8277

Mason County Mental Health
Office
701 Viand St.
Point Pleasant, WV 25550
(304) 675-2361

Wayne County Mental Health
Office
Wayne County Health
Department
Wayne, WV 25570
(304) 272-3466

Lincoln County Mental Health
Office
6990 State Route No. 3
West Hamlin, WV 25571
(304) 824-5790

Center on Alcoholism and Drug
Abuse
40 12th St.
Wheeling, WV 26003
(304) 233-8700

Skyline Hospital
Box 648
White Salmon, WV 98672
(509) 493-1101

Sundown M. Ranch Corporation
Box 81
White Swan, WV 98952
(509) 874-2520

Wisconsin

Memorial Medical Alcohol and
Drug Treatment Center
522 7th Ave. West
Ashland, WI 54806

Rock County Alcohol and Drug
Abuse Unit
Box 351
Janesville, WI 53545
(608) 752-9481

Family Counseling Center of
Kenosha County, Inc.
1202 60th St., Suite 115
Kenosha, WI 53140
(414) 657-6187

Kenosha Memorial Hospital
6308 8th Ave.
Kenosha, WI 53140
(414) 656-2011

Unified Counseling Service
Box 351, Route 2
Lancaster, WI 53813
(608) 723-7430

Psychiatric Nursing Intervention
Clinic
University of Wisconsin
Hospitals
1300 University Ave.
Madison, WI 53706
(608) 262-3116

Counseling Center of Milwaukee,
Inc.
2390 N. Lake Dr.
Milwaukee, WI 53211
(414) 271-4610

Meta House
2571-2579 N. Farwell Ave.
Milwaukee, WI 53202
(414) 962-4024

A-Center
2000 Domanik Dr.
Racine, WI 53404
(414) 632-6141

Waukesha Memorial Hospital
725 American Ave.
Waukesha, WI 53186
(414) 544-2244

Lutheran Social Services
903 2nd St.
Wausau, WI 54401
(715) 842-3343

Dewey Center
1220 Dewey Ave.
Wauwatosa, WI 53213
(414) 258-4094

Wyoming

Northern Wyoming Mental
Health Center
900 W. 6th St.
Campbell, WY 82716
(307) 682-4762

Central Wyoming Counseling
Center
504 S. Durbin St.
Casper, WY 82601
(307) 237-9583

Well Being
837 East C
Casper, WY 82601
(307) 265-9555

Western Wyoming Mental
Health Center
132 No. Glenwood
Jackson, WY 83001
(307) 733-2046

Southeast Wyoming Mental
Health Center
Ivanson Memorial Hospital
Laramie, WY 82070
(307) 745-7015

Southeast Wyoming Mental
Health Center
215 E. 21st St.
Torrington, WY 82240
(307) 532-4211

Self-Help Organizations

SELF-HELP activities are not a new phenomenon. Supportive assistance is the essence of strong neighborhoods and of religious, service, and social groups. However, since the 1950s, the growth of these caring peer groups into membership organizations has been extraordinary. Theorists have written many tracts in search of explanations. Some of the theories make particular sense, especially for women. Research has shown that in 1976 and 1977 sixty national organizations relating to women were formed because "no service was available in response to their particular problematic condition."

Another explanation for this rapid growth is the desire for community with compatible others who share a similar position. Especially because the stigmas attached to alcoholism, drug dependency, mental illness, or physical handicaps produce subtle and overt alienation, the support, help, and companionship of empathetic people are greatly needed. Support groups keep growing because they meet human needs. Even those professionals who direct medical detoxification programs supplement their therapy with outside, noninstitutional support groups. Patients become members and, finally, helpers.

Personal success through group processes does require a high degree of involvement. One must be willing to help others and to accept help. Those who benefit most characteristically grow to new levels of competence both within and outside the group structure.

The ideologies of self-help organizations tend to be fixed. Although the format of local meetings may deviate in order to accommodate the needs of the membership, the substantive teachings are structured. Certain groups' purposes were once conveyed by their names: Narcotics Anonymous, Alcoholics Anonymous, Widow-to-Widow, Women for Sobriety, Other Victims of Alcoholism, Families Anonymous, Parents-Without-Partners, and so on. Increasingly these organizations have expanded from single-problem identification to encompass the collateral needs of their respective members. Self-destructive behavior may be caused by, or may result from, another stressful condition or relationship, and so the goals of recovery must include treatment of the broader dimensions of debilitation. Therefore, whatever the immediate symptoms to be remedied, a helping group, whose principles are consistent with the new member's values where kinship is likely, may provide strength and growth for multiple needs.

In addition to the groups identified and the known location of current meeting places, please take the time to seek other programs, local or national. Through state and municipal agencies, through the women's centers at universities or colleges, or in phone book listings, there is help available for our endangered species.

Arizona

Families Anonymous

367 N. 21st Ave.
Phoenix, AZ
(602) 258-8512

1719 E. Prince Rd.
Tucson, AZ
(602) 326-6115

Narcotics Anonymous
St. Luke's Hospital
525 N. 18th St.
Phoenix, AZ 85006
(602) 258-7373

California

Addicts for Christ
Garden Grove, CA
(714) 839-6961
Contact: Rev. Able Rivera

Alcoholics Anonymous

123 W. Windsor Rd.
Glendale, CA
(213) 242-1350

423 E. Angeleno Ave.
Burbank, CA
(213) 843-0618

4343 Redford Ave.
Studio City, CA
(213) 769-8755

Families Anonymous
Box 344
Torrance, CA 90501
(213) 775-3211

11435 Downey Ave.
Downey, CA 90241
(213) 775-3211

1611 E. Sycamore
El Segundo, CA 90245
(213) 775-3211

Pacifica House
13515 S. Vermont
Gardena, CA

Orange County Mental Health
17055 Newland St.
Huntington Beach, CA

Families Anonymous (continued)

15151 Cordova
La Mirada, CA 90638
(213) 775-3211

1228 Pine Ave.
Long Beach, CA

3507 W. Beverly Blvd.
Los Angeles, CA 90004
(213) 775-3211

1730 W. Vernon Ave.
Los Angeles, CA 90062
(213) 775-3211

Trinity Lutheran Church
1001 W. Rowell/11th St.
Manhattan Beach, CA

11027 Burbank Blvd.
North Hollywood, CA 91601
(213) 775-3211

401 S. Tustin Ave., Rm. 204
Orange, CA 92666
(213) 775-3211

Open Door - Switchboard
714 A Deep Valley Dr.
Palos Verdes, CA

1680 N. Fair Oaks Ave.
Pasadena, CA 91103
(213) 775-3211

786 N. Garey Ave.
Pomona, CA 91767
(213) 775-3211

8995 Magnolia Ave.
Riverside, CA 90503
(714) 688-9500

1221 Ocean Ave.
Santa Monica, CA 90401
(213) 775-3211

Church of Christ
11935 Wick Ave.
Sun Valley, CA

18646 Oxnard St.
Tarzana, CA 91356
(213) 775-3211

Families Anonymous (continued)

3250 Lomita Blvd.
Torrance, CA 90505
(213) 775-3211

1423-A Marcelina
Torrance, CA 90501
(213) 775-3211

3812 Sepulveda Blvd., Rear
Torrance, CA 90501
(213) 775-3211

Girl Scout House
Columbia Park, High St.
Turlock, CA

15520 Sherman Way
Van Nuys, CA 91406
(213) 775-3211

520 S. Larkellen
West Covina, CA 91790
(213) 775-3211

Hope House
7382 Garden Grove Blvd.
Westminster, CA

E. Whittier Presbyterian Church
14061 E. 2nd St.
Whittier, CA

Family Services of Long Beach
16704 Clark Ave.
Bellflower, CA 90705
(213) 867-1737

Family Services Association of
Long Beach
1041 Pine Ave.
Long Beach, CA 90813
(213) 436-9893

Harbor Community Involvement
1111 Figueroa Pl.
Wilmington, CA 90744
(213) 830-8603

La Clinica Libre Del Puerto
1020 East L St.
Wilmington, CA 90744
(213) 830-0100

Marriage and Family Counseling
44848 N. Cedar
Lancaster, CA 93534
(805) 948-0871

Nar-Anon Family Groups
Group Headquarters
Box 2562
Palos Verdes Peninsula, CA
90274

Nar-Anon
Prince of Peace Church
Fremont Blvd.
Fremont, CA

6170 Thornton Ave.
Newark, CA

1710 Moorpark (Corner of
Leigh)
San Jose, CA

1625 Franklin Ave.
Sonoma County Drug Abuse
Santa Rosa, CA

Narcanon U.S.
6425 Hollywood Blvd.
Suite 206
Hollywood, CA 90028
(213) 469-8347

Narcotics and Alcoholics
Anonymous
641 Shalimar St.
Costa Mesa, CA 92627
(714) 642-9373

Narcotics Anonymous
World Service Office
Headquarters
Box 622
Sun Valley, CA 91352

18252 Arrow Highway
Azusa, CA 91702
(213) 388-0225

Box 76
Berkeley, CA 94701

2220 Ceader St. (church) at
Spruce St.
Berkeley, CA

Narcotics Anonymous (continued)
1800 South C St.
Oxnard, CA 93030
(213) 388-0225

16635 Paramount Blvd.
Paramount, CA 90723
(213) 388-0225

1680 N. Fair Oaks Ave.
Pasadena, CA 91103
(213) 681-2575

2600 Middlefield Rd.
Fair Oaks Community Center
Redwood City, CA

8 Sun St.
Salinas, CA

California and Taylor Streets
Grace Cathedral Library Room
San Francisco, CA

90 - 9th St., near Mission St.
San Francisco, CA

240 Turk St.
San Francisco, CA

80 S. 5th St.
Lower Floor
San Jose, CA

Newport and Pine
San Jose, CA

Community General Hospital
Mental Health Center
San Luis Obispo, CA

Parents United
Fellowship Hall
Orange, CA

Project Jove II
812 N. Fair Oaks Ave.
Pasadena, CA 91103
(213) 793-2151

Self-Help Center
1436 E. Huntington Dr.
Duarte, CA 91010
(213) 358-0107

The Alcoholism Center for
  Women, Inc.
1147 S. Alvarado St.
Los Angeles, CA 90006
(213) 381-7805

La Casa de las Madres
Box 15147
San Francisco, CA 94115
(415) 626-9337

The Woman's Alliance
1509 E. Santa Clara Ave.
San Jose, CA 95116
(408) 251-5522

Ocean Park Community Center
245 Hill St.
Santa Monica, CA 90405
(213) 399-9228

San Diego Widowed to Widowed
  Program, Inc.
6655 Alvarado Rd.
San Diego, CA 92120
(714) 280-5467

Women's Educational
  Preparation Training
333 S. Los Angeles St.
Los Angeles, CA 90013
(213) 627-5781

River Queen Women's Center
17140 River Rd.
Guernewood Park, CA 95446
(707) 869-0333

YWCA of Sonoma County
Box 3506
Santa Rosa, CA 95402
(707) 546-9922

The Sacramento Women's
  Center, Inc.
1230 H St.
Sacramento, CA 95814
(916) 446-2791

The Center for Feminist Therapy
  and Education, Inc.
944 Market St., Suite 209
San Francisco, CA 94109
(415) 397-2023

Woman's Resource Center
1105½ S. Hill St.
Oceanside, CA 92054
(714) 722-1606

Colorado
Families Anonymous
St. Luke's Church
2000 Stover
Ft. Collins, CO

Delaware
Narcotics Anonymous
1225 Market St.
Wilmington, CA

Georgia
Families Anonymous
  Covenant Presbyterian Church
  2126 W. Edgewater Dr.
  Albany, GA

  Clubhouse: Clubhill Apt.
  3728 Armour Ave.
  Columbus, GA

Narcotics Anonymous
De Kalb Addiction Center
1260 Briarcliff Rd., N.E.
Atlanta, GA 30306

Northside Alcoholics Benevolent
  Association (NABA)
1809 Briarwood Rd.
Atlanta, GA 30329
(404) 636-8044

Alcohol and Drug Abusers
  Pulling Together (ADAPT)
(404) 378-3627 or 231-1422

Hawaii
Narcotics Anonymous
2611 Ala Wai Blvd.
Honolulu, HI 96815

Maui Women's Counseling
Center (clinic)
Maui, HI

Alternatives for Women
YWCA
Oahu, HI

AA Wahine Meeting
Oahu, HI

Idaho
Families Anonymous
YMCA
8th and Washington
Boise, ID

Volunteers in Service to
Substance Abuse (VISA)
Department of Health and
Welfare
Bureau of Substance Abuse
508 E. Florida St.
Nampa, ID 93651
(208) 466-8981

Illinois
Families Anonymous
Chicago, IL
(322) 848-9090

Our Savior's Lutheran Church
1234 N. Arlington Heights Rd.
Arlington Heights, IL

Family Counseling Service
411 W. Galena
Aurora, IL

Gateway House Foundation
2403 E. 75th St.
Chicago, IL

Maze One
3126 N. Broadway
Chicago, IL

Benton Community Settlement
3052 S. Gratten
Chicago (Bridgeport), IL

Forest Hospital Professional
Center

Families Anonymous (continued)
1717 Rand Rd. (Route 12)
Des Plaines, IL

Group for Newcomers
Forest Hospital, 4th Floor
Auditorium
555 Wilson Lane
Des Plaines, IL
(312) 848-9090

First Presbyterian Church
17929 Gottschalk
Homewood, IL

First Christian Church
1826-16th St.
Molino, IL

First United Church
931 Lake
Oak Park, IL

St. Paul's Cathedral
3601 N. North St.
Peoria, IL

High School
N. Chaffer
Roxana, IL

American International
Hospital
Shiloh Blvd.
Zion, IL

Indiana
Narcotics Anonymous
c/o Common Ground Center
310 E. Court Ave.
Jeffersonville, IN 47130

Iowa
Families Anonymous
First Congregational Church
608 W. 4th St.
Waterloo, IA

Kansas
Carriage House Project
1100 Gage St.
Topeka, KS 66604
(913) 273-4141

Families Anonymous
540 N. Main St.
Wichita, KS

Narcotics Anonymous
Central Kansas Foundation for
Alcohol and Chemical
Dependency
112½ N. Santa Fe
Salina, KS 67401
(913) 825-6224

Kentucky
Families Anonymous
Southfield's
Anchorage, KY

Community Center
6108 Bardstown Rd.
Ferncreek, KY

Methodist Church
3600 Tater Creek Rd.
Lexington, KY

Parents Anonymous
c/o YWCA
2000 E. 20th St.
Owensboro, KY 42301

Maryland
Addicts Anonymous
Education Building
St. Mark's United Presbyterian
Church
10701 Old Georgetown Rd.
Bethesda, MD 20014

Families Anonymous
Woodlawn Senior High School
1801 Woodlawn Dr.
Baltimore, MD

St. Luke's Episcopal Church
Old Georgetown Rd. and
Grosvenor Lane
Bethesda, MD

Michigan
Families Anonymous
Federal Savings & Loan

Maple Hill Mall, W. Main St.
Kalamazoo, MI

Minnesota
The Bakery
2603 Bloomington Ave. South
Minneapolis, MN
(612) 348-4166

Black Women's Program
2104 Stevens Ave. South
Minneapolis, MN
(612) 871-2360

Chemical Abuse Service
Agency — CASA
203 Prescott
St. Paul, MN
(612) 227-0831

Chrysalis
2104 Stevens Ave. South
Minneapolis, MN 55404
(612) 871-2603

Drug Abuse Services Project
1900 Chicago Ave. South
Minneapolis, MN

Families Anonymous
Growth Center
Brainerd, MN

Biltmore Motel (Cavalier Rm.)
5212 Vernon Ave. South
Edina, MN

St. James Church
2028 - 7th Ave. East
Hibbing, MN

Pharm House Crisis Center
1911 Pleasant St.
Minneapolis, MN

The Storefront
6612 Lyndale Ave. South
Minneapolis, MN

St. Peter's Catholic School
2620 N. Margaret St.
North St. Paul, MN

Families Anonymous (continued)
Prescott House
203 Prescott
West St. Paul, MN

Indian Neighborhood Club
1805 Portland Ave. South
Minneapolis, MN
(612) 871-1925

Metropolitan Institute on Black
Chemical Abuse
3010 - 4th Ave. South
Minneapolis, MN
(612) 827-4611

Minneapolis YWCA
1130 Nicollet
Minneapolis, MN

On Top (Chemically Dependent
Mothers)
2104 Stevens Ave. South
Minneapolis, MN
(612) 874-8611

St. Stephen's Guild Hall
2211 Clinton Ave. South
Minneapolis, MN
(612) 870-0559

Mississippi
Narcotics Anonymous
184 Longino St.
Jackson, MS
(601) 968-1108

Singing River Drug Treatment
Program
4507 McArthur St.
Pascagoula, MS 39567
(601) 769-1793

Missouri
Families Anonymous
Jefferson Barracks, Building #25
VA Hospital
St. Louis, MO

Montana
Southwestern Montana Drug
Program
1539 - 11th Ave.
Helena, MT 59601
(406) 449-2827

Nebraska
Families Anonymous
Southminster Methodist Church
2915 S. 16th St.
Lincoln, NE

Narcotics Anonymous
Pius X Grade School
6905 Blondo St.
Omaha, NE
(402) 477-1336

New Jersey
Families Anonymous
J. Runnels Hospital, Rose Hall
Plainfield Ave.
Berkeley Heights, NJ

New Mexico
Families Anonymous
St. Marks on the Mesa
430 Dartmouth N.E.
Albuquerque, NM

New York
Access
401 Main St.
Islip, Long Island, NY
(212) 281-6694

Baden St. Drug Center
30 Vienna St.
Rochester, NY 14605

Boces Drug Abuse Prevention
Program
6820 Thompson Rd.
Syracuse, NY 13211
(315) 437-1631

Camelot
263 Richmond Ave.
Staten Island, NY 10302

Families Anonymous
31 Linden St.
Brooklyn, NY

Christian Science Church
W. 83rd St.
New York City, NY

Schenectady, NY
(518) 895-2362

John 3:16 Center
115 Lyell Ave.
Rochester, NY 14608

Project Create
108 W. 112 St.
New York, NY 10036

North Carolina
Families Anonymous
St. Martin's Episcopal Church
1510 E. 7th St.
Charlotte, NC

North Dakota
Narcotics Anonymous
St. Joseph's Hospital
7th St. West
Dickinson, ND 58601
(701) 225-6771

United Hospital — North Unit
1200 S. Columbia Rd.
Grand Forks, ND 58201
(701) 775-9791

Ohio
Families Anonymous
Christian Family Center
4014 Glenway Ave.
Cincinnati, OH 45205
(513) 921-2945

Cleveland, OH
(216) 321-1920

Methodist Church
771 E. 260th St.
Euclid, OH

Narcotics Anonymous
Holy Name Church

McMillan and Auburn Avenue
Cincinnati, OH 45219
(513) 281-3991

Oklahoma
Families Anonymous
8100 N.E. 23rd St.
Oklahoma City, OK
(405) 232-6844

Mid-Del Youth and Family
Center
4501 S.E. 28th St.
Del City, OK 73115
(405) 670-1478

Narcotics Anonymous
Community House
421 N.E. 14th St.
Oklahoma City, OK
(405) 232-1937

Tulsa, OK
(918) 584-4592

Pennsylvania
Confront Inc.
1130 Walnut St.
Allentown, PA 18102
(215) 433-0148

Diagnostic and Rehabilitation
Center
304 Arch St.
Philadelphia, PA 19106
(215) 925-3909

Families Anonymous
Family Counseling Clinic
603 W. Main St.
Bloomsburg, PA

TRW — Conference Room
601 E. Market St.
Danville, PA

Brushtown Athletic Association
Clubhouse
RD #4, Route 116
Hanover, PA

Families Anonymous (continued)
First Presbyterian Church
Green Lane and Emilie Rd.
Levittown, PA

First Baptist Church
S. Third St.
Lewisburg, PA

St. Matthews Episcopal Church
Front St. and Woodlawn Ave.
Sunbury, PA

YMCA Building
High and Chestnut Streets
West Chester, PA

H.A.N.A.
Box 653
New Cumberland, PA 17070
(717) 737-6242

Keenan House
114 N. 9th St.
Allentown, PA 18102
(215) 439-8479

Mr. Penn Group
Faith Lutheran Church
25th and Filbert Streets
(210 N. 25th St.)
Mt. Penn, PA 19606
(215) 582-1753

Narcotics Anonymous
First Presbyterian Church
4th and Market Streets
Bloomsburg, PA
(717) 784-7154

Holy Spirit Hospital
5 E.N. 21st St.
Camp Hill, PA

Church of the Brethren
West and Walnut Streets
Carlisle, PA

Old Airport Hanger
Stanley St.
Chambersburg, PA

Grove Presbyterian Church
330 Bloom St.

Narcotics Anonymous (continued)
Danville, PA
(717) 275-7651

One Day at a Time Group
R.D. #5, Clinic Rd. off
Route 11
Danville, PA
(717) 275-2751

United Methodist Church
Blakely St.
Dunmore, PA
(717) 343-7189

United Methodist Church
1501 Derry St.
Harrisburg, PA

Box 1521
Kingston, PA 18704
(717) 344-9527

First Baptist Church
51 S. 3rd St.
Lewisburg, PA
(717) 524-9973

6261 N. Broad St.
Philadelphia, PA 19141
(215) 276-2703

Immaculate Conception School
Taylor and Olive Streets
Scranton, PA
(717) 344-9527

St. Andrews Episcopal Church
Foster and Frazier Streets
State College, PA
(717) 237-8353

St. Matthews Episcopal Church
Front and Woodlawn Streets
Sunbury, PA
(717) 286-7521

810 Club House
First and Campbell Streets
Williamsport, PA
(717) 322-9142

Annunciation Church
4th and Walnut St.
Williamsport, PA
(717) 323-6397

Narcotics Anonymous (continued)
Divine Providence Hospital
Grampian Blvd.
Williamsport, PA
(717) 326-6734

Wyoming Borough Building
Wyoming, PA
(717) 829-3446

Women for Sobriety, Inc.
Box 618
Quakertown, PA 18951
(215) 536-8026

Juniata Valley Tri-County
Drug and Alcohol Program
27 W. Market St.
Lewiston, PA 17044
(717) 242-1446

South Carolina
Narcotics Anonymous
Morris Village
Alcohol and Drug Addiction
Center
610 Faison Dr.
Columbia, SC 29203
(803) 758-4154

South Dakota
Families Anonymous
Ben French Station
Black Hills Power and Light
Deadwood Ave.
Rapid City, SD

Tennessee
Joseph W. Johnson, Jr. Mental
Health Center, Inc.
Moccasin Bend Rd.
Chattanooga, TN 37405

Texas
Families Anonymous
Church of the Heavenly Rest
602 Meander
Abilene, TX

Webbs Chapel Methodist
Church

Families Anonymous (continued)
2536 Valley View Lane
Dallas, TX

St. Stephan's Episcopal Church
1603 Ave. J (Student Center)
Huntsville, TX

7th and Olive Streets
Longview, TX

Friends Anonymous
Temple, TX
(817) 773-5483

Program for Alcoholism,
Addictions, Stress and Anxiety
(PAASA)
3501 Mills Ave.
Austin, TX 78731
(512) 452-0361

Utah
Narcotics Anonymous
Alcohol Recovery Center
667 E. South Temple
Salt Lake City, UT 84103
(801) 328-0023

Northwest Multipurpose Center
1300 W. 3rd North
Salt Lake City, UT 84116

Recovery, Inc.
(801) 268-2402
(For information and literature)

Washington
Narcotics Anonymous
First Congregational Church
1220 N.E. 68th St.
Vancouver, WA

409 E. 16th St.
Vancouver, WA
(206) 696-1751

Urban Indian and Alcohol and
Drug Component
c/o Volunteer Services
Box 1809
Yakima, WA 98907

Wisconsin

Families Anonymous

Eau Claire, WI
(715) 834-4986

459 E. First St.
Fond du Lac, WI

Our Saviors Lutheran Church
612 Division St.
La Crosse, WI

Good Shepherd School
N. 81 W. 17658 Christman Rd.
Menomonee Falls, WI

109 E. Keefe
Milwaukee, WI

DePaul Hospital
4143 S. 13th
Milwaukee, WI

Narcotics Anonymous
Dewey Center Milwaukee
  Psychiatric Hospital
Treatment for Chemical
  Dependency
1220 Dewey Ave.
Wauwatosa, WI 53212
(414) 258-2600